Breast Massage

Debra Curties, R.M.T.

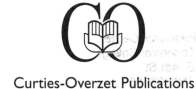

Curties-Overzet Publications

Figures 12,15,17, 20, and 22 are reprinted with permission from: Hughes L.E., Mansel R.E., Webster D.J.T., **Benign Disorders and Diseases of the Breast,** *Baillière Tindall,* ©1989

Figures 11,16, 23, and 24 are reprinted with permission from: Cawson R.A., McCracken A.W., Marcus P.B., Zaatori G.S., **Pathology: The Mechanisms of Disease,** *2nd ed., C.V. Mosby Co.,* ©1989

Figure 14 is reprinted with permission from: Kumar V., Cotran R.S., Robbins S.L., **Basic Pathology,** *W.B. Saunders,* ©1997

Figures 13,18, and 19 are reprinted with permission from: Powell D.E., and Stelling C.B., **The Diagnosis and Detection of Breast Disease,** *C.V. Mosby Co.,* ©1994

Figure 2 is reprinted with permission from: Haagensen C.D., **Diseases of the Breast,** *3rd ed., W.B. Saunders,* ©1986

Breast Massage
Debra Curties, R.M.T.
© Copyright 1999

To order copies, please contact:
Curties-Overzet Publications Inc.
330 Dupont Street, Suite 400
Toronto, Ontario
Canada M5R 1V9
Toll Free Phone: 1-888-649-5411
Fax: 416-923-8116
Website: www.curties-overzet.com
E-mail: info@curties-overzet.com

National Library of Canada Cataloguing in Publication

Curties, Debra (Debra Vivian), 1953-
  Breast massage / Debra Curties.

Includes bibliographical references and index.
ISBN 0-9685256-1-X

  I. Title.

RM721.C87 1999   618.1'90622   C99-018005-0

Acknowledgements

I would like to thank Pam Fitch for your collaboration and support as a colleague, and for those gentle pushes when needed. Without your help this book might still be a work in progress.

Thanks to Ellen Prose for your advice and support, and for your excellent photography. Also to Bev Ransom for the beautiful illustrations and all your technical help in putting the pieces of the book together. And to Jerry Overzet for your tremendous support and assistance in making things happen at the business end.

My warmest appreciation to Frances Farquhar, Renate Mohr, Kim Ostrom, Trish Dryden, Christine Laflamme-Snow, Giselle Sehault, and Pat Madden for your generous support and participation and your belief in the value of this project.

As always, thank you to the people of Sutherland-Chan School, who nurture and support me in all my endeavours.

An Open Letter to Massage Therapy Students

Dear Student,

I have on many occasions been asked to explain why we make breast massage a mandatory part of the massage therapy training program at our school. You may or may not be studying at a school which requires you to learn breast massage - you may already be a practising therapist as you read this - but I would like to explain why I believe that breast massage should be taught as an integral part of the training to become a massage therapist.

Breasts are body tissues with their own health needs. At some point in time, most women will experience breast congestion, breast pain, discomforts of diagnostic or surgical procedures, and anxieties about lumps or other changes in their breast tissues. Pregnancy and breastfeeding have their own set of associated breast tissue needs. Unfortunately, many women experience physical and psychological trauma related to their breasts. And there is breast cancer - it impacts directly on the lives of many women, and indirectly on all of us.

Conditions and occurrences affecting breasts lead women to seek medical help and to self medicate. Statistics indicate that many women complain of breast pain to their doctors. At the same time most sources reporting these stats believe that women underreport breast problems, presumably for similar reasons to those which lead us to be uncomfortable about breast massage.

The fact that breasts are strongly associated with sexual touching and attractiveness does not mean that they cannot or should not receive health care. In fact, this symbolism adds a set of psychoemotional concerns that many women need help with in order to feel more at ease about doing routine self examination and seeking the therapies they need in a matter-of-fact way.

The multidimensional significance of breasts means that health care practitioners involved with breast health must be carefully trained. We need to be able to deal with the significance and sensitivity involved in touching breasts; we need to be able to communicate clearly; and we need to know how to maintain good professional boundaries. In our school, we work to meet this mandate by instructing in draping and privacy issues, techniques which are best to use and to avoid, how to talk about breast massage, how to conduct the consent dialogue, when to refer to another massage therapist, and all the other factors that go into having a completely professional approach.

I cannot ascribe to the thinking that by examining or treating a breast (with consent) a trained health care practitioner is by definition doing something sexual. A therapist with sexual or abusive intent can convey this in the way he or she touches any body part, and with all manner of other verbal and non-verbal cues. The well intentioned therapist will be especially conscious of avoiding any such possible interpretations when treating body parts known to be more emotionally charged. We assume that doctors, nurses, lab technicians and others can appropriately handle the necessities of working with breast tissues. Are massage therapists different?

Massage therapy is effective 'wellness' treatment for breasts because they particularly need good circulation and tissue mobilization for optimum health. Poor circulation can produce various uncomfortable symptoms. Breast scarring, which is more common than we often realize, can cause painful syndromes and obstruct blood and lymph flow. Some believe there may be a correlation between chronic poor breast drainage and susceptibility to malignancy. Massage techniques and hydrotherapy may in fact turn out to be some of the most effective modalities for addressing such problems and promoting breast health.

Many women need more help becoming comfortable with breast self examination than they receive in their doctors' offices. Some have traumatic histories and need assistance achieving a sense of normalcy about their breasts and the types of touch involved in seeing to their care. As well, a skilled palpator may be more successful in picking up early stage breast tissue changes needing medical follow-up than a client would herself. Given the time spent, the regular treatment intervals, the privacy of the circumstances, and the trained empathy and physical skill of the practitioner, massage therapists really have something to offer.

There are some very important safety concerns, both for the client and the practitioner. Some people have histories which can make it difficult for them to distinguish present realities from past experiences, and some people find it especially tough to talk clearly about what they accept and cannot accept as treatment. I am referring to both client and health care worker here. Our personal stories are often the same. There are no magic answers about how to identify the situations to avoid. Most of the confirmed discipline cases I am aware of have arisen from circumstances where the massage therapist did not communicate clearly, did not properly obtain consent, and/or did not maintain professional boundaries. However, there are some definite risks - there are high risk clients and there are high risk circumstances. It is important to keep in mind that these circumstances are not exclusive to breast massage. Getting a good basic education, finding a peer support group or a skilled supervisor once out in the field, and pursuing advanced training in specialized areas of treatment and client interaction are important safeguards.

In Ontario, a guideline has been put in place to support client and therapist protection. Breast massage is not considered an automatic part of a standard full body massage. It has been categorized as a special treatment which must be specifically consented to by the client. Arguments can be made for and against this stance, but it is helpful, given the controversies about touching breasts, to have a guideline which recognizes that it is not safe for therapists to make the assumption that clients will automatically consider breast massage part of what they are requesting when they seek massage treatment.

Can we justify letting our concerns about risks cause us to completely overlook the legitimate treatment needs of breasts? Is it right that breast health care is not getting the attention from our profession that it should? Should women have to suffer from pain and other symptoms that could be ameliorated if we were comfortable addressing them in the way we would be for other body tissues? Is there any way that massage therapists can help in the fight against breast cancer? These are important questions, and it is our duty as members of the professional health care community to give them serious thought. Breast massage will not be right for every client and every therapist, but are we doing our best to fulfill our profession's obligations? Are we wrestling in a principled way with the dilemmas involved or are we putting our heads in the sand?

I hope I have explained why we include breast massage in the massage therapy curriculum at our school. We try to find non-traumatizing ways to help students with individual needs and concerns to meet this program requirement. We do not always get everything right, and we have had lots of student/teacher/administration discussions about how to improve the training. But through working at it with dedication, we are finding that our students are much more capable and comfortable with breast massage and its related skills than they were in the past.

I also hope that this book will make a contribution to your learning and help promote the use of breast massage, where appropriate, as part of the fundamental set of health care services we provide for those who choose massage therapy.

Debra Curties, RMT

WOMEN TALK ABOUT BREAST MASSAGE BENEFITS

One of the things that we often forget, when we become focused on the discomforting issues that breast massage raises for us, is that it can have real and important benefits for our clients...

Debra C.

I start with a story of my own because it is often experiences as a client that nurture my faith in the efficacy and value of massage and re-motivate me as an educator. A few years ago I had a painful deep biopsy in one of my breasts. It happened rapidly after one of those scary 'found a lump' scenarios; almost before I had time to think I was in the OR. Fortunately, it was found to be an irregularly shaped cyst and I knew in my head that I was all right. The incision had gone straight down through my breast, which was bruised, hard, and swollen, and had a fair bit of nerve irritation. Two weeks later there wasn't much relief and I still hadn't thought about getting breast massage (you tell me why). In the third week I booked an appointment, asking for breast massage and neck work, since my neck was also sore from the intubation. Within five minutes of the beginning of the treatment I felt the sense of frozen apprehension begin to leave me, and as the treatment progressed I could feel my neck, shoulders, and jaw let go of a terrified holding I wasn't really conscious was still stuck in my body. The first breast massage was simple and soothing; after this first session my symptoms improved by about 50%. Four breast treatments in three weeks were enough to restore normal softness and circulation to the breast tissues and healing proceeded quickly and uneventfully.

Liz B.

There was a time when I couldn't imagine anyone ever touching my breasts, let alone massaging them. Now I feel the massage isn't complete unless my whole body is touched - arms, legs, breasts, belly, back, neck and head.

Yvonne L.

After treatment for breast cancer, my right breast felt hard and lumpy. The doctor said it would always feel that way because of the radiation. But after receiving only three breast massage treatments the breast feels almost the same as the other one. The hardness is gone. It really made a difference.

Bev H.

After breast reduction surgery, I was left with a line of tension near the bottom scar. Raising my arms over my head caused painful pulling and stretching along the length of the scar. Breast massage has really helped alleviate the pressure. The scar doesn't bother me at all now.

Fran F.

I find breast massage is valuable to me in two ways. The first is my practical reason: since I have lost 24 lymph nodes on one side, I know that breast needs assistance with lymph drainage. The other is my emotional reason: it's so reassuring to me to have another set of professional hands working with my breasts. It's comforting to know that another professional who is knowledgable about breast tissue is checking for any changes, especially since I have numb areas where the surgery was done.

Brenda D.

Once when breastfeeding my first child, I developed a blocked duct. It was extremely painful and uncomfortable. I am a massage therapist, and I massaged the breast until the blockage cleared. When the duct finally released, milk sprayed clear across the room.

Christine W.

I was diagnosed several years ago with fibrocystic breasts. I find I need regular massage to keep my breast tissue soft and malleable. When I go without breast massage, the lumpiness and discomfort soon return.

Renate M.

I had my first breast massage two and a half months after a full mastectomy. It was really noticeable to me that massage loosened up the whole area and made the tissue feel more 'normal'. The treatment also really helped with range of motion. Even after just one treatment I had a lot more mobility raising my arm. Emotionally, it was very helpful to have someone else touch the 'new' tissue area to help me reclaim it as part of my body, a part that needs love like all the other parts.

Diane McG.

I have fibrous breasts which were always very sore and engorged premenstrually. They were feeling like that the day we learned breast massage in school. I volunteered to be the 'demo', and so I received a treatment from the teacher. I was amazed at how effective it was - I could feel fluid moving and clearing in my breast. Since then I have made a practice of getting regular breast massage and doing self massage almost daily. I have virtually no problems with breast soreness now.

Alice E.

I had a breast massage the day before I was to see my oncologist. My massage therapist gave me a thorough treatment and reassured me that my breasts felt normal...no lumps and bumps. I sailed into my oncologist's office full of confidence and for the first time in several years I didn't feel afraid of what he might find.

Outline

ISSUES, DECISION-MAKING, AND GUIDELINES FOR THE MASSAGE THERAPIST

HOW TO DO BREAST MASSAGE

Learning Objectives

The purpose of this book is to support the broader use of breast massage through contributing to the education and skill of massage therapists. Massage therapy can be an important and effective treatment approach for breast tissues. It can also assist women with comfort issues related to having their breasts seen and touched, engaging in routine breast health care practices like self examination, and overcoming other types of fears and obstacles.

Breast tissues have therapeutic needs like other tissues, but given the complexities of societal symbolism and the personal associations breasts have for all of us, providing breast massage is not a simple matter of proper use of technique.

In the course of reading this book, the reader will develop:

1. an overview of the design, structure, and functions of the tissues of the breast, including its relationship to nearby structures and its circulatory and neural supplies

2. an understanding of the indications and contraindications for breast massage

3. an appreciation of the life cycle changes breasts experience and their specific needs in different cycles

4. a basic knowledge of conditions commonly found in breasts

5. the ability to identify ominous signs

6. guidelines and techniques for draping breasts and performing breast massage

7. an appreciation of the self awareness, sense of boundaries, and professionalism required of the massage therapist who provides breast massage

8. greater comfort in talking about breast massage with clients and in obtaining clear and thorough consent to treatment

9. an appreciation of when not to offer breast massage and when to refer to another practitioner

10. a set of guidelines to support the safety needs of the client and the practitioner

11. a level of comfort and confidence which makes it possible to offer competent and effective breast treatment when appropriate

Key Words

mammary

pertaining to the breast or tissues of the breast

mast-

prefix which means pertaining to the breast or breast tissues

mastalgia

breast pain; also sometimes called mammalgia or mastodynia

mastitis

breast inflammation and/or infection

mastectomy

full or partial removal of a breast, usually because of cancer; radical mastectomy refers to removal of the whole breast and ipsilateral lymph nodes

implant

breast implants are surgically placed prostheses, usually soft capsules containing saline solution or silicone, which are used to increase breast size or to reconstruct or otherwise standardize breast shape and appearance

lump

a non-specific term used in the breast context to mean a palpable density, nodularity, mass, or other distinct structural change in the feel of a breast's tissues

involution

1. the monthly process which ensues when a pregnancy has not occurred; the breasts recede from a state of readiness for pregnancy and lactation

2. the return to pre-pregnancy state after breastfeeding ends

3. regression and resorption of the breast alveoli and duct structures which begins at approximately age 35 and is completed following menopause; caused by hormonally directed changes in the woman's reproductive system

lactation

the period in which a woman's breasts are producing milk and she is breastfeeding an infant

cyst

cysts are encapsulated sacs filled with fluid or semi-fluid substances; they can occur throughout the body, including in breasts

discharge

the term used to describe fluid seepage from a nipple, especially in circumstances where the woman is not pregnant or breastfeeding

ominous signs

in the breast context, used to mean signs or symptoms which are suggestive that cancer could be present and should therefore receive further investigation

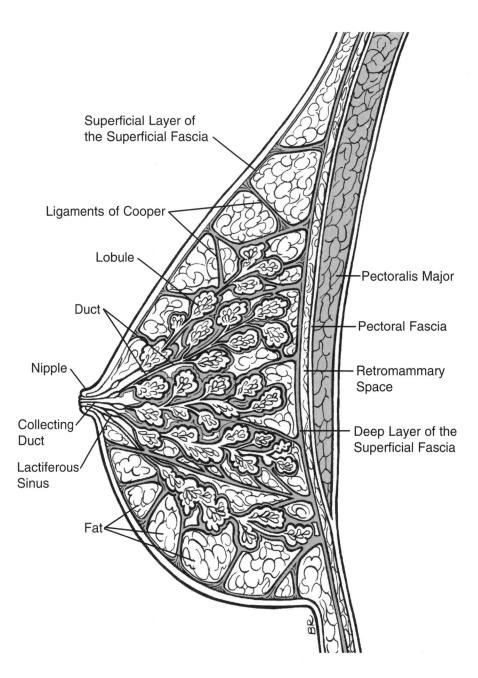

Superficial Layer of
the Superficial Fascia

Ligaments of Cooper

Lobule

Duct

Nipple

Collecting
Duct

Lactiferous
Sinus

Fat

Pectoralis Major

Pectoral Fascia

Retromammary
Space

Deep Layer of the
Superficial Fascia

Figure 1. The female breast

ANATOMY AND FUNCTION OF THE BREAST

Breast Anatomy

The breast is a specialized gland structure which evolves essentially as an appendage of the skin. It develops within the layers of the subcutaneous superficial fascia. The most superficial of these fascial layers is positioned directly under the skin and forms the anterior boundary of the mammary gland. The deepest layer forms the posterior boundary and sits over the muscles of the chest wall. The tissues which make up the breast lie in between, anchored by extensions of these fascial membranes known as ligaments of Cooper or Cooper's Ligaments. These thickened fascial strands extend into the breast to provide a supporting framework. Cooper's Ligaments are also called the suspensory ligaments. They are illustrated in Figure 1 on the opposite page.

Deep to where the breast attaches to the posterior layer of the superficial fascia is a zone of loose areolar tissue called the retromammary space. The arrangement of loose connective tissue in this 'space' allows the breast to move fairly freely over the fascia covering pectoralis major. The retromammary space also plays a very important role in the lymphatic drainage of the breast, as we will discuss shortly.

The rounded contour of the breast projects anteriorly from the chest wall and suspends loosely against gravity. There are no muscles or cartilaginous structures within the breast, so it relies on its fascial envelope and suspensory ligaments for integrity and support. This information is important for the massage therapist, who should avoid techniques which could unduly stress or stretch these structures.

In the centre of the breast's surface is a circle of darker skin called the areola. While usually a somewhat deeper version of the woman's skin colour, the areola can become very darkened in high estrogen states like pregnancy. The skin of the areola contains a large number of specialized sebaceous glands, referred to as Montgomery's glands, which are clearly visible as small bumps.

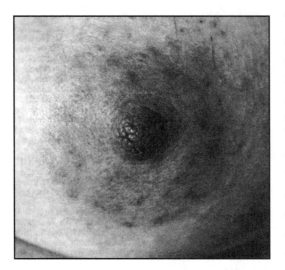

The nipple is positioned at the centre of the areola. Both the sub-areolar tissue and the nipple are richly supplied with smooth muscle which runs in both circular and radiating patterns. When these muscle fibres contract the nipple erects, and if the woman is lactating, the milk sinuses empty. The nipple is also a centre of sexual sensation and is served by a large number of sensory nerve endings.

Figure 2. Normal presentation of the nipple and areola
(Haagenson C.D., Diseases of the Breast, 3rd ed., W.B. Saunders, ©1986)

Breast Tissue Boundaries[1]

Most of us are not aware that women have more breast tissue than is evident from observing the breast's rounded contour. The typical boundaries of the visually apparent breast are as follows:

upper:	2-3rd rib
lower:	6-7th costal cartilage
medial:	sternal edge
lateral:	anterior axillary line

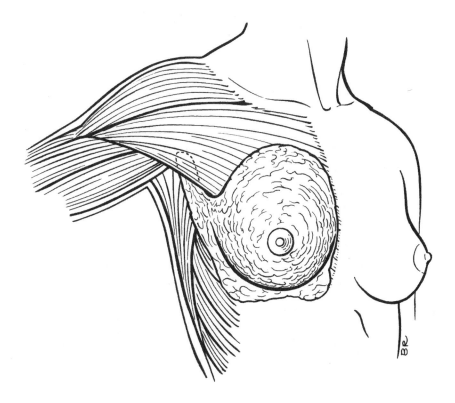

Figure 3. Breast tissue extends well beyond the breast contour

What is unclear on routine observation is that thin layers of mammary tissue reach beyond these borders, extending to:

upper:	lower edge of the clavicle
lower:	1" or so below the breast contour, overlying upper fibres of rectus abdominis
medial:	sternal mid-line
lateral:	anterior edge of latissimus dorsi variable amount of breast tissue continuing into the axilla

Look closely at Figure 3 to compare the protuberant breast contours (left breast) with the boundaries of mammary tissue as shown on the right side. This information about the actual extent of breast tissue is very important to the practitioner because findings of breast tissue tenderness, nodularity, and benign and malignant lumps may all occur in this larger zone beyond the contours of the breast. These thin extended layers may also swell painfully with inflamed or engorged breasts.

The breast overlies several muscles. On average 50% of the breast sits over pectoralis major, and the rest over the other muscles of the chest wall, especially serratus anterior. Variable small amounts of breast tissue overlie latissimus dorsi superolaterally, and the lower edge covers a bit of rectus abdominis.

It is common and quite normal for a woman's two breasts to be different sizes. The most common breast abnormality is presence of one or more accessory nipples, usually found along the 'nipple line' in the abdomen. Another frequently occurring breast irregularity is a greater than average extension of breast tissue into the axilla. It is important to be aware of this anomaly because it can look like a mass. (See Figure 4.) The tissue will not appear ominous in that it is malleable, its boundaries are soft and easily palpated, and it moves well in relation to nearby tissue. Doctor examination is necessary, however, to ensure that the formation is simply extra breast tissue.

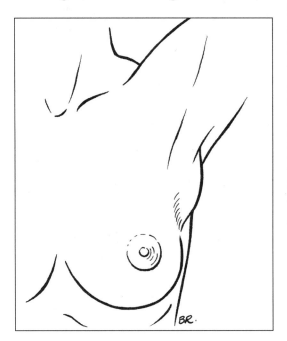

Figure 4. Extra mammary tissue in the axilla

Quadrant System of Breast Tissue Landmarking

For purposes of landmarking and recording, the breast tissues are usually charted using the map illustrated below. This quadrant system is widely used to communicate locations of tissues, structures, and lesions within the breast.

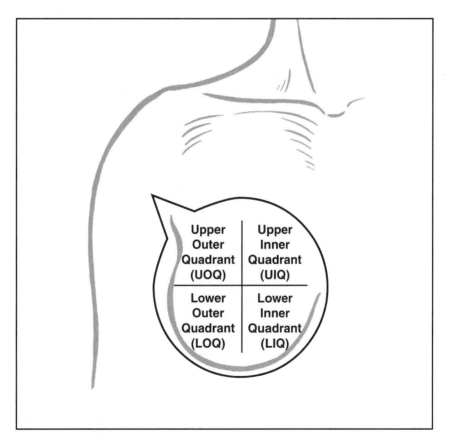

Figure 5. System used to identify tissue locations within the breast

Microanatomy and Function

Although the massage therapist does not need highly detailed knowledge of breast microanatomy, some understanding is useful, particularly in relation to the development and progress of conditions seen commonly in clinical practice, and to assist in the selection of the most effective techniques when massaging.

The large fascial layers mentioned in the previous section provide the structural framework, or stroma, of the breast. The parenchyma, or functional tissue, is a glandular system of 15-20 lobes responsible for producing and delivering milk to the nursing infant. Each lobe contains milk producing cells organized into structured clusters called lobules, and a duct system to propel the fluid they produce toward the nipple. Lobes are separated from each other and their neighbour tissues by thick connective tissue capsules which create a boundary between the internal and external environments of each lobe.

The rounded form of the breast depends more on fat than on its functional tissue. Fat is the 'filler' which encases and insulates the lobes. Distribution of fat is greater in the upper two quadrants. The upper half of the breast, particularly the upper outer quadrant, also contains more glandular tissue and is therefore more dense.

The design of the 'glandular field' of the breast has many similarities to the respiratory unit in the lung. Each lobe has its own collagen membrane capsule on which sit numerous glandular epithelial cells. These cells are arranged so that they face into a collecting space. Since they are secretory cells this arrangement provides for collection of the fluid they produce. The basement membrane under the cells assumes rounded shapes, creating a cluster design. Each loop in the cluster is called an alveolus or acinus (both names are commonly used). There

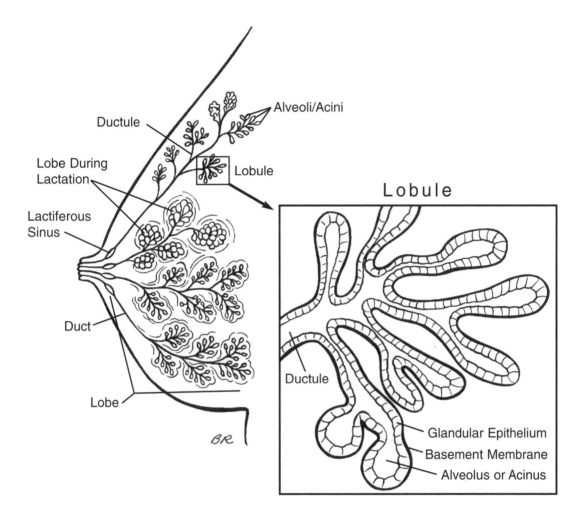

Figure 6. The breast parenchyma

are, on average, 10-100 alveoli/acini in a lobule and 20-40 lobules in a lobe. The lobule is considered the basic functional unit of the breast. Refer to Figure 6 for an illustration of these structural relationships.

Each lobule empties into its own ductule. These ductules in turn propel their contents into the central duct channel of their lobe. In this way milk produced in the alveoli can be moved in the direction of the nipple. The duct system of each lobe terminates in a reservoir called a milk sinus (lactiferous sinus) located behind the nipple.

The cells lining the alveoli and ducts are laid down in two layers. Specialized epithelial cells capable of contraction, called myoepithelium, lie under the glandular cells at the exit areas of the acini and along the walls of the ducts. When these cells contract, the fluids in the acini are pushed into the small ductules, and then along the duct channels. The myoepithelial cells are not innervated by nerves; the stimulus must be hormonal.

The breast's system of ducts is surrounded by loose areolar connective tissue, which creates a soft and flexible type of stroma. The lobe structure, comprised of the three dimensional lobules surrounded by connective tissue and serviced by small blood and lymphatic vessels, looks like a sponge when seen in cross section.

The Breast's Circulation

Blood Supply

The breast contains no muscles, nor other connective tissues except its fascial stroma, so the primary physiological aims of breast massage relate to enhancing circulation and drainage. Both the arterial and venous blood supplies of the breast are susceptible to compression from musculoskeletal structures, and to reduced circulation when shoulder and thorax mobility are decreased.

Arterial Supply:
Arterial blood is supplied to the breast by the subclavian artery, via several of its main branches (most importantly the axillary, internal mammary, and intercostal arteries). The subclavian artery is a large central vessel and its branches are responsible for delivering fresh blood to both the medial and lateral aspects of the breast.

Venous Drainage:
The venous drainage system of the breast originates from a rich venous plexus deep to the areola. Small local veins and their branches

follow essentially the same pathways as their companion arterial vessels. Venous blood from the breast drains primarily to the internal mammary and axillary veins. See Figure 7.

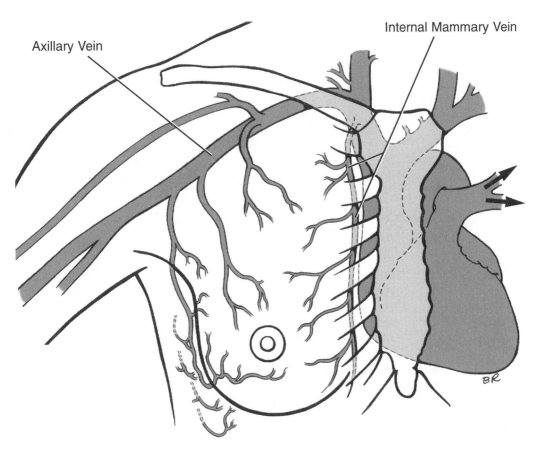

Axillary Vein

Internal Mammary Vein

BR

Figure 7. Veins which drain the breast

Breasts Get TOS Too!

Thoracic outlet syndrome, a common compression syndrome which affects the axillary/subclavian vessels (and the brachial plexus) can impair circulation to and from the breast to a significant degree. Many practitioners are not aware that this condition can result in pain, numbness, and tingling affecting the breast as well as the upper limb.

Lymphatic Drainage

The lymph system, which clears substances from the intercellular spaces in tissues, is considered the most important factor in breast tissue drainage. It is widely speculated that chronic impairment of lymph drainage may be implicated in many breast health problems, including cancer. Cancer metastasis routes through lymphatic channels result in the most ominous types of breast cancer spread, leading one to wonder how significant the effectiveness and resilience of the lymph drainage system may be in the prevention or control of breast cancer. From the massage therapist's point of view, understanding the design of the breast's lymphatic drainage is essential for effectiveness of treatment.

The breast's skin surface, the areola, and the nipple are all richly supplied lymphatically. As well, large numbers of tiny lymphatic vessels run through the loose areolar connective tissue surrounding the lobules and their ducts, thereby draining the breast parenchyma. These small vessels are generally believed to be valveless[2,3]. Their valvelessness is significant because it means that drainage along these intrinsic channels can be adversely affected by gravity, especially in large pendulous breasts. It also means that they can easily become ineffective when there is obstruction from scars, swelling, or other forms of compression.

Drainage from the microvessels servicing the various breast structures converges on several plexi, which empty into larger collecting channels to carry the lymph from the breast.

While one might naturally assume that superficial lymph vessels would drain superficially and the more in-set ones through deeper channels, in fact, most lymph flow in the breast is from superficial to deep[4]. This is consistent with the general pattern of drainage for skin and subcutaneous tissue. The significance of this information is that a high percentage of breast-generated lymph, carrying assorted potentially irritating and pathogenic substances, must be carried back through the breast tissue to the retromammary space before it accesses external draining vessels. Recognizing this anatomical fact is crucial for the massage therapist - without it one might intuitively select surface focused drainage techniques destined to have limited effectiveness.

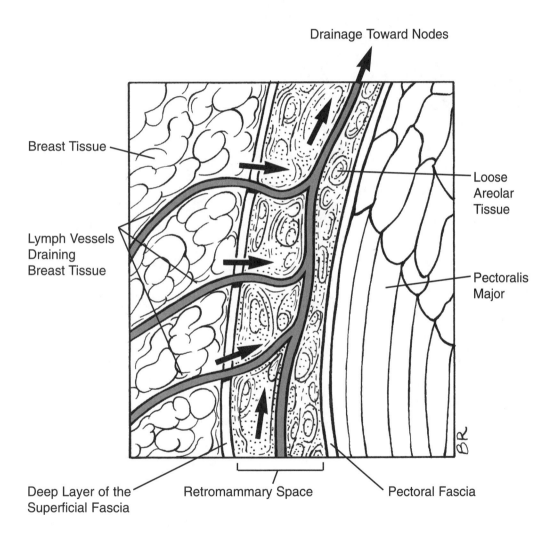

Figure 8 illustrates the drainage of lymph posteriorly from the breast via the retromammary space. Compression of this space can significantly reduce clearance of lymph from the breast.

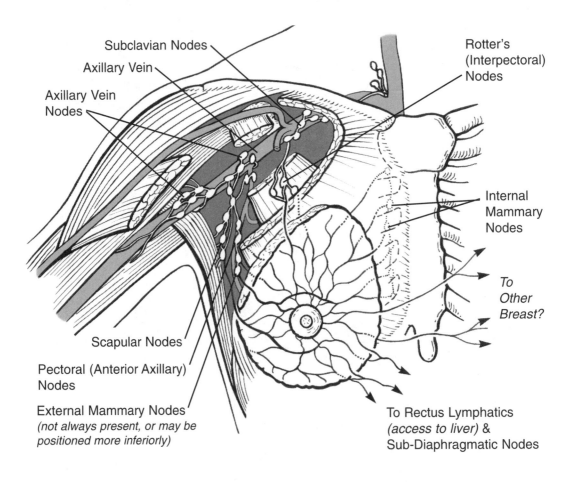

Figure 9. Lymphatic drainage of the breast

Eventually all breast lymph drains into regional nodes, the majority of which are in the axilla. These nodes are filled with immune system cells and are responsible for filtering the lymph and destroying organisms and other undesirable substances it may contain. Discrepancies exist in the reporting of amounts of lymph clearance to different nodal groups. This may suggest that women are individually different. The reader is referred to Figure 9 for illustration of the groups of nodes most significant in breast drainage.

In general, it can be stated that in the vicinity of 75% of breast lymph goes to the system of nodes in the axilla, with most of the remainder draining toward the internal mammary chain[5]. Small amounts of drainage move in the direction of the rectus abdominis lymphatics and the subdiaphragmatic nodes. Some authors acknowledge the presence of drainage channels between the two breasts, citing the frequency of metastasis in this pathway, while others deny finding such channels on dissection.

There is also a small amount of lymph drainage through the intercostal spaces to the posterior paravertebral nodes. Some of the medial breast is cleared by lymphatics accompanying the perforating internal thoracic blood vessels to drain into the internal thoracic group of nodes in the thorax, and then on into the mediastinal nodes.

Lymph flow en route to the axillary drainage system passes through a series of node clusters which in turn drain toward major nodes lying alongside the axillary and subclavian veins. All of these pathways can be adversely affected by compressive and postural restrictions. One set of nodes, called the external mammary nodes, lies in many women beneath the lateral edge of pectoralis major, in the vicinity of the serratus anterior digitations. A significant set of interpectoral nodes (called Rotter's nodes) is situated between pectoralis major and minor. These channels can be especially affected by injuries, tension, or shortening of the involved muscles.

While the axilla's node system is clearly of great consequence, the importance of the internal mammary route cannot be underestimated[6]. The vessels in this route must travel through pectoralis major; drainage may be impaired by tension of this muscle medially.

Another highly significant finding is that the major nodal groups do not drain specific zones of the breast[7]. Although most lymph clearance will tend towards the closest group of nodes, Turner-Warwick found "no striking tendency for any particular quadrant to drain in one direction"[8], reporting for example that the internal mammary nodes receive lymph drainage from both the lateral and medial halves of the breast. This information seems particularly useful to the manual therapist because it suggests that inefficient or obstructed drainage (e.g. by scar tissue) might be successfully redirected through other channels.

Do Bras Promote Breast Cancer?

One study has concluded that there may be a breast cancer risk associated with bra wearing, especially wearing one more than 12 hours a day, and wearing it for sleeping. In an interview study involving 4,730 Caucasian American women, half of whom had breast cancer and the other half of whom had no history or indication of the disease, the researchers asked the subjects about their bra wearing habits and history. Nearly twice the number of women with cancer reported that their bras had consistently left red marks or caused skin irritation. 18% of the women in the breast cancer group as compared to 3% in the control group had the habit of wearing a bra to bed. The researchers, Ross Singer and Soma Grismaijer, postulated based on their statistics that limiting bra wearing to under 12 hours a day may decrease breast cancer risk by as much as 19%. Another major concern is wearing bras that are too small or otherwise too tight. Many women do not take note of the fact that their bra size is expected to increase several times in their lifespan.

Singer and Grismaijer have published their findings in a book titled *Dressed to Kill: The Link Between Breast Cancer and Bras* (Avery Publishing Group, 1996). Singer indicated in an interview with the Valley Advocate in Hatfield, Massachusetts, that they believe the problem is chronic compression of lymphatic drainage channels caused by holding the breast pressed back against the chest wall and constricting natural drainage-promoting mobility of breast tissue.

This study has not been duplicated and the findings remain controversial, but they are interesting in light of how the breast drainage system is designed anatomically.

The Breast's Nerve Supply

Nerves acting within the breast are principally somatic sensory nerves. Generally speaking, the areola and nipple are richly supplied while the rest of the breast is not. This means that while the nipple and areola are acutely sensitive to pain and other sensations, breast tissue in general is less so. The rich nipple innervation provides the basis for the sucking reflex and reflexes causing uterine contraction. Nipple sensation is also strongly associated with the sexual response.

Sensory nerve supply to the superior aspect of the breast is via the supraclavicular nerves (C3, C4). The medial and lateral aspects are serviced primarily by branches of the thoracic intercostal nerves, many of which must penetrate through pectoralis major to reach their supply tissues. Authors vary on which and how many intercostal nerves are responsible for these functions - nerves 2-5 may all be involved. A major supplier of the upper outer quadrant is the intercostobrachial nerve (C8, T1), which sends a large branch to the breast as it passes through the axilla. The responsibilities of nerves supplying the breast do not include any servicing of its glandular function, all of which is under hormonal control[9]. Autonomic nervous system involvement appears to be restricted to sympathetic innervation of blood vessels.

As will be discussed in a later section, a percentage of breast pain comes from musculoskeletal origins. This means that it is important for the massage therapist to be aware of the possibilities of compression, irritation, and damage to nerves which innervate breast tissues. The most clinically relevant locations are the axilla, the upper intercostal spaces, and pectoralis major, whose involvement can lead to nerve branch compression in several locations. Brachial plexus and cervical nerve root compression can also result in breast pain.

Changes During Pregnancy and Lactation

The pregnant woman's body undergoes high levels of hormonally directed growth and metabolic activity and the breasts are very much part of this process. They progress through several stages of change and development toward the ultimate goal of providing nourishment for the baby after it is born. These stages of preparation for breastfeeding are for most women accompanied by periods of soreness and congestion.

In the first trimester, emphasis is on growth of new ducts and early formation of new lobules. By 5-8 weeks into the pregnancy breast enlargement is significant. Dilation of superficial veins, increased pigmentation of the nipple/areola, and tissue 'heaviness' are all typical.

In the second trimester, the focus is on lobule formation and glandular cell activation. Alveolar epithelium converts into more specialized secretory cells with surface microvilli. Colostrum, a milk precursor, begins to appear in the alveoli. Hypertrophy of myoepithelial cells occurs in preparation for the work of mobilizing milk through the duct passageways. There is also an increased presence of connective tissue and fat.

Breast tissue activity is intense in the first half of pregnancy - milk supply can be adequate with early delivery of 16 weeks onward. Women usually experience their greatest breast tenderness in the second through fourth months. While the degree of discomfort varies, for many women the tenderness in their breasts is quite marked during this period. In addition to soreness, frequently the breasts also feel hot and painfully congested.

In the last trimester, there are increases in glandular cell number and development, further addition and dilation of acini, and more production of colostrum. By the end of the pregnancy there has been a significant increase in the volume of parenchyma relative to other breast components. In the second half of pregnancy overall breast size also continues to increase. An average woman's breast will weigh 200 grams pre-pregnancy and 400 grams at term. In addition, there will be an increase of 180% in mammary blood flow[10]. In the third trimester, the woman's breasts are not so much tender as they are heavy and achy.

The hormonal influences on the breast tissue change with the birth, transforming the epithelial cells into a fully secretory state. From birth to 4-5 days postpartum the breasts enlarge substantially, initially producing a volume of colostrum, then milk. They are usually quite tender at this time. Nipple soreness is also common at the beginning of breastfeeding and usually persists until the areolar skin becomes accustomed to the unusual use. Tissue breakdown may occur and can lead to bacterial mastitis, a condition we will discuss later.

As breastfeeding proceeds, the breasts are again experienced as more heavy and achy than actually sore. Vascularization continues to be high, and the feeling of hot, uncomfortable congestion can be present. However the routines of lactation, once established, usually result in norms of breast filling and emptying (and of skin tissue acclimatization) that are comfortable for most mothers. In Figure 10 you can see the appearance of the breasts of a lactating mother who has a 3 month old infant.

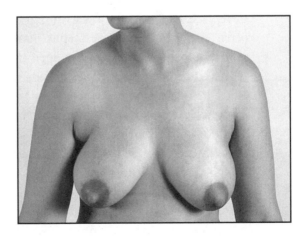

Figure 10. The appearance of lactating breasts

Discontinuing breastfeeding results in stoppage of milk production and regression of the additional breast parenchyma that has been put in place. This process takes some time and usually involves several days to a few weeks of congested distension. The resulting discomfort can often be ameliorated by massage and hydrotherapy.

Changes With Age - Involution

The term **involution** is used to describe changes occurring in the breast parenchyma which are a regression away from readiness for pregnancy and lactation. For example, the breast is said to involute in the second part of the menstrual cycle following an ovulation which has not resulted in conception. As has just been mentioned above, breast tissue also involutes at the cessation of breastfeeding.

In a larger context, involution is also the term used to describe the changes occurring from 35 years of age onward, as the breasts begin the slow process of replacing their functional tissues with fat. Both lobular parenchymatous structures and supportive fascial stroma are eventually converted; the resulting post-menopausal breast is almost entirely comprised of fatty tissue. This process proceeds slowly. It involves passing through various stages, including an intermediate one of replacing lobe structures with dense collagen. The deposited fibres often entrap and compress epithelial cells. Over time the collagen regresses to be replaced by fat deposition. Involution of the lobules may result in tiny microcysts, a stage which is considered normal.

These changes, occurring primarily in the years from 35 to 60, are significant in that they give rise to many of the conditions referred to as benign breast disease. Examples include formation of dense nodular areas in the breast tissue and development of macrocysts. Some, previously considered disorders, are now believed to be completely normal aspects of the involution process. Others, while not exactly normal, are commonly seen variations and not considered dangerous[11]. Considerable research attention has been directed in the last two decades to better determination of what is and is not ominous, since most benign and malignant breast changes coincide in the 40 to 60 age range.

Many of the tissue changes associated with involution of the breasts through perimenopause and menopause are symptom free; others involve general soreness, local tenderness, or other discomforts. The supplanting of the stroma by fat also explains the more pendulous posture of the older woman's breast.

CLINICAL INFORMATION FOR THE MASSAGE THERAPIST

Introduction

Most women these days experience intense and deep-seated fear about the possibility of finding anything abnormal in their breasts. Added to the general fearfulness, and perhaps because of it, some women completely avoid regular medical and self examination. Massage therapists are in the interesting position of being considered knowledgeable professionals without being strongly associated with anxieties about medical procedures and diagnoses.

One of the challenges facing us in massage therapy is to become knowledgeable enough about the range of normal, benign, and ominous formations in the breast to be able to play a responsible role in palpating clients' tissues and communicating about what we are feeling. The massage therapist does not diagnose, and should always refer a woman to her physician when something new is identified. However, clients often want our help in monitoring their breasts, and many seek to engage in further discussion about what they have been told by a doctor.

It is also important for the massage therapist not to feel undue apprehension about breast palpation or to induce such a state in the client. In the anxious atmosphere that prevails, a practitioner who acts or speaks in ways which could be interpreted as foreboding may cause totally unnecessary traumatization of clients. Many massage therapists readily admit that they are not confident in their knowledge of common breast tissue formations, and feel torn between a need to make sure that something ominous is not overlooked and the desire to have calm and comfort in the breast massage treatment.

The data which follows about the common benign conditions should help by giving basic information about how they appear clinically and how they typically feel on palpation. Information will also be provided about ominous symptoms and palpatory signs. It is important to keep in mind that benign conditions sometimes mask cancer or unexpectedly become cancerous, while very ominous signs can turn out to have a completely benign causation. Sometimes one practitioner will pick up on something that another, palpating on a different day or from a different vantage point, will not notice. Nothing can take the place of a good routine of medical monitoring. Our role is in fact to support that routine.

Common Benign Breast Conditions (ANDI)

The terms 'benign breast disease' and 'fibrocystic breast disease', although still widely used, are falling into disfavour. In the past, virtually all new tissue formations were considered potentially dangerous and surgical removal was the norm. This was especially true if the woman was experiencing uncomfortable symptoms like pain, or if there was a family breast cancer history. Research and clinical surveys have increasingly shown, however, that breast symptoms do not correlate well with histological findings, and that progression to more advanced disease is not typical in most common conditions. One group of scientists has declared fibrocystic breast disease "a non-disease"[12].

While women do suffer in large numbers from breast pain and other symptoms, current experts are questioning the previously held view that most of the causes are in some way pathological and potentially ominous. It is also true that many commonly experienced symptoms do not originate in the breast at all; the prevalence of external sources of mastalgia, for example trigger points, is becoming more common knowledge.

Understandable confusion also arises from the fact that cyclical and reproductive processes, as well as the processes involved in involution, generate a broad range of tissue change. Changes associated with involution become apparent by age 35. This means that menstrual cycles, reproduction, and involution can run in tandem for 15-20 years, involving a great deal of tissue transformation and increasing the possibility of aberrations from normal. Women taking the birth control pill show a smaller incidence of benign breast disorders, indicating that cyclical hormonal fluctuations play a significant role in their development[13].

It appears likely that most benign breast tissue aberrations arise because of imbalances in levels of estrogen and progesterone, or altered target tissue sensitivity to these hormones[14]. The imbalances can be relatively small. Various theories, for example, inherited tendency and responses to stress, have been put forward to explain these minor deviations. Given that the hormonal imbalances generally occur within what is considered normal ranges, it could be said that medical knowledge is not yet refined enough to detect and interpret such shifts. Yet they may over time lead to alterations in tissues which step outside of what is considered normal formation. As a result, defining the border between 'normal' and 'pathological' is difficult.

In the past ten years the trend has been toward de-pathologizing many conditions. While causal relationships are still in doubt, clinical studies have helped clarify the likelihood of various common tissue changes leading to more serious disease. A new term, Aberrations of Normal Development and Involution (ANDI), is increasingly being used. The conditions placed under the ANDI heading confer very small or no added cancer risk and are so common as to not really merit the label of pathology or disease[15].

The massage therapist researching this subject will find that authors vary greatly in their use of new and old terminologies. Similarly, doctors may use a range of terms in discussing benign breast conditions with their patients. Further questions may be necessary if you encounter terms like 'fibrocystic breast disease' or 'mammary dysplasia', which are not very clear or specific.

A List of Common ANDI

1. Fibroadenosis

The term fibrosis refers to overgrowth of stromal elements. As has already been mentioned, deposition of collagen fibres is a normal stage of lobe replacement in involution. In some women these changes occur outside of involution or begin earlier than expected. The term adenosis denotes overgrowth of glandular epithelium, and is often referred to as 'epithelial hyperplasia'. It results in enlargement of lobules beyond the average of 10-100 alveoli. Most types of adenosis are very common and not considered dangerous, although there are a few atypical variations that may be pre-cancerous and need careful monitoring.

Because these two aberrations often occur together, they are frequently named fibroadenosis. Fibroadenosis is a condition of the premenopausal breast. Estimates of its incidence range between 30-100% of women in the 20-45 age group[16]. Occurrence is greatest in the outer half of the breast, especially the upper outer quadrant. It is usually bilateral, with one side being more affected than the other for most women.

Fibroadenosis is also sometimes called 'painful nodularity'. On palpation it feels like a nodular region which is more firm and uneven than the nearby tissue. It does not have clear edges or feel like a discrete lump; rather it seems like an irregular dense zone within the standard breast tissue arrangement. It is usually sensitive to palpation, although the degree of sensitivity varies. For most women fibroadenosis becomes noticeably more tender in the second half of the menstrual cycle and less so again after the menstrual period is over.

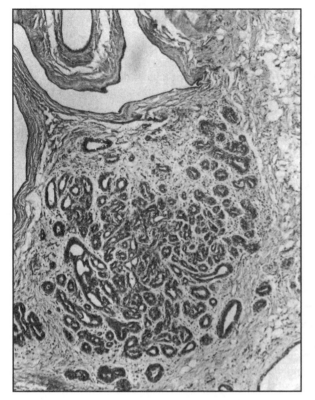

As with most ANDI conditions, fibroadenosis is believed to be caused either by an imbalance in the hormones which control breast tissues or by an abnormal response of sections of breast tissue to normal hormonal influences. Women who have anovulatory cycles are less likely to suffer from fibroadenosis[17], suggesting a clear relationship to cyclical hormonal stimulation. Stress may be implicated in fibrosis, and caffeine consumption is also believed by some researchers to play a role, although there are mixed findings on this and the theory does not have broad support.

Figure 11. Histological view of fibroadenosis (*Cawson R.A., McCracken A.W., Marcus P.B., Zaatori G.S., Pathology: The Mechanisms of Disease, 2nd ed., C.V. Mosby Co., ©1989*)

2. Fibroadenoma

Fibroadenoma is a condition of lobular overgrowth. The result is "a discrete benign tumour showing evidence of connective tissue and epithelial proliferation"[18]. It is common and easily diagnosed by its clinical features. The mass is round or lobulated, feels smooth, 'rubbery', firm, and discrete, and is highly mobile relative to the adjacent tissue. It is surrounded by its own fibrous capsule and typically crowds and compresses nearby breast tissue. Calcification may occur within the tumour structure and may be palpable as a much more 'hard' section of the mass.

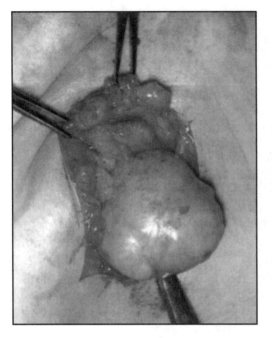

Fibroadenomas are generally seen in young women age 16-30. When found in older women they are still assumed to have originated at this age. They are slightly more prevalent in the left breast. There is an initial growth phase (1-5 years) after which the tumour size usually remains static at 1-3 cm. in diameter. It often regresses gradually. Growth beyond 5 cm. would be considered atypical and merit further exploration.

Figure 12. The typical fibroadenoma of adolescence (Hughes L.E., Mansel R.E., Webster D.J.T., Benign Disorders and Diseases of the Breast, Baillière Tindall, ©1998)

Although discovered less commonly in women 35 or older, fibroadenomas when found at this stage are often less mobile due to involutional fibrous changes in the nearby tissue. They also tend to lose their characteristic surface smoothness, and because of the increased cancer risk in this age group, will often be biopsied to ensure correct diagnosis. Fibroadenomas usually involute in perimenopause to be replaced by fibrous tissue. They may occasionally be discovered in the elderly where they appear as small hard masses which have a high degree of mobility.

It is estimated that 10-25% of women have one fibroadenoma or more[19]. The cause is not known, but the fact that lobular proliferation occurs in response to estrogen stimulation suggests that a fibroadenoma may arise as the result of a lobule becoming unusually estrogen responsive. Fibroadenomas usually enlarge rapidly during pregnancy[20], further suggesting an estrogen connection. It has also been noted that fibroadenomas may be more common in young women with menstrual irregularities.

Since this condition is not typically painful and is benign and self-limiting in the vast majority of cases, it is usually left untreated.

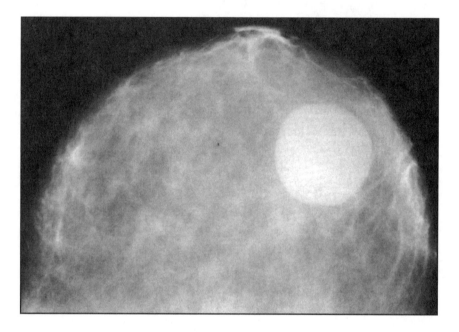

Figure 13. Fibroadenoma appearance on mammogram (*Powell D.E. & Stelling C.B., The Diagnosis and Detection of Breast Disease, C.V. Mosby Co., ©1994*)

3. Sclerosing Adenosis

Sclerosing adenosis produces enlargement of lobules, via marked epithelial proliferation, so that they come to contain many more alveoli than average. Myoepithelial overgrowth and considerable fibrosis also occur. What is seen on histological examination are bands of fibrous tissue surrounding hyperplastic epithelium, compressing it into small distorted islands of ductal and acinar cells (see Figure 14). The infiltration of ducts by glandular cells and collagen fibres may be so extensive that their lumina are eliminated.

The tissue shows signs of both proliferative and involutional aberrations, making it more likely to be a condition arising from a distorted combination of both processes. This conclusion is reinforced by the fact that sclerosing adenosis is almost never seen in women under 30.

On palpation, sclerosing adenosis feels like a poorly defined mass of firm fibrous tissue which has a degree of hardness more similar to carcinoma than the other ANDI mentioned. It usually has an irregular surface and may present as a dense core surrounded by softer lobulated areas. Its degree of firmness and its irregular features mean that the mass must be carefully examined to ensure that it is not a malignancy. Despite superficial similarities to breast carcinomas, however, sclerosing adenosis carries minimal risk of proceeding to become cancerous.

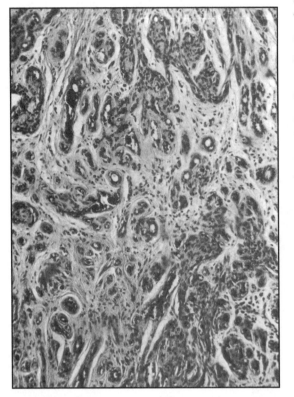

Figure 14. Histological view of sclerosing adenosis
(Kumar V., Cotran R.S., Robbins S.L., Basic Pathology, W.B. Saunders, ©1997)

The proliferating epithelial cells frequently invade nerves and blood vessels. This causes pain in about 50% of cases. The structure can also attract calcium deposition in a way which adds to the pain experienced by some women. There is also the possibility of secretory changes which may result in a milky type of nipple discharge.

Although common, the incidence of sclerosing adenosis is not well documented; one study reports it as a finding in 7-20% of biopsies[21]. Sclerosing adenosis is rarely treated medically, except at times for pain.

4. Cysts

Microcysts are considered a normal aspect of lobular involution. Each acinus becomes a small cystic structure as a stage in the resorption of its

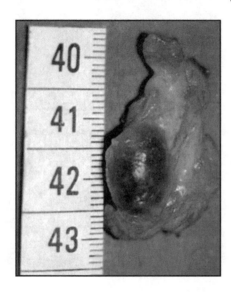

glandular cells. For unknown reasons believed to be hormonally based (perhaps with familial tendency), a certain percentage of women develop a larger type of cyst, most accurately referred to as a macrocyst. It represents most or all of a lobule which has failed to undergo a well integrated involution process. In the past, breast cysts were believed to be precancerous, but they are currently categorized in the ANDI group of conditions. Several large careful studies have shown lack of significant increased risk of cancer development due to the presence of a cyst[22].

Figure 15. A typical breast macrocyst   (Hughes L.E., Mansel R.E., Webster D.J.T., Benign Disorders and Diseases of the Breast, Baillière Tindall, ©1998)

The macrocyst appears to result, at least in part, from obstruction of the lobule's exit into its ductule. The lumen obstruction is likely caused by involution-based cell changes and/or by collagen deposition. There may be kinking of the ductule due to fibrous changes in the surrounding stroma. Fluid dynamics in the lobule may also be a factor, with loss of the balance normally occurring between fluid production and resorption. The macrocyst is a dilated fluid-filled sac derived from what was once a lobule and attached to the lobe tree by the fibrous remains of the lobule's ductule. In fact, several of a lobe's lobules may become cystic; groupings of cysts in one location are the norm. This can create a 'grape cluster' appearance.

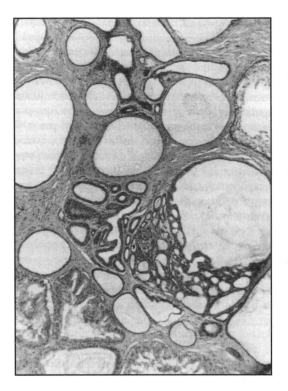

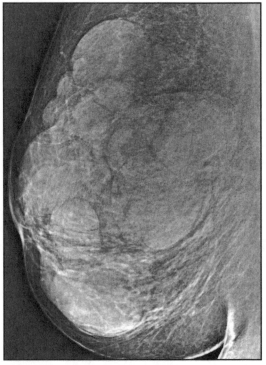

Figure 16. Breast macrocysts viewed histologically. Note the region of fibroadenosis.

(Cawson R.A., McCracken A.S., Marcus P.B., Zaatori G.S., Pathology: The Mechanisms of Disease, 2nd ed. C.V. Mosby Co., ©1998)

Figure 17. Mammogram showing a breast with multiple macrocysts.

(Hughes L.E., Mansel R.E., Webster D.J.T., Benign Disorders and Diseases of the Breast, Baillière Tindall, ©1998)

The obstruction of the ductule may be complete, incomplete, or reversible. This may explain why cysts can fluctuate a great deal in fluid content, and at times completely resolve. These changes in cyst behaviour are poorly understood.

Most of the time cysts are fairly lax and therefore blend into the feel of the breast tissue. This can make them hard to palpate, especially if they are not superficial. However, rapid changes in cyst fluid content are common - when a cyst becomes tense with fluid it can quickly become palpable.

Palpable macrocysts appear as rounded, oval, or lobulated smooth discrete lumps which move well with the surrounding tissue on circular palpation. The term which characterizes the palpatory feel of a cyst is 'fluctuant'. Because of the fluid content, the palpator can cause changes in the contour of the lump, much like gently pushing on the surface of a balloon filled with water. However, some cysts will be quite tense and have a more solid feel. The single palpable cyst is usually part of a cluster, the majority of which are softer or deeper and cannot be felt. Cysts may or may not be tender to palpation. Larger cysts may also become visible when the woman lies supine.

Macrocysts are generally found in women 35-55. There is no relationship between age and number or size of cysts. They disappear rapidly after menopause, although they may be seen in older women taking hormone supplementation. It is important to note that the appearance of a macrocyst five years or more after menopause in the woman not on hormone replacement therapy is cause for concern. In this instance they are often manifesting as part of the development of a carcinoma.

Occurrence of cysts is typically bilateral, with statistically slightly greater distribution in the left breast. They are usually found in the upper quadrants; two thirds occur in the UOQ. There is considerable variation in the statistics about how common macrocysts are. One autopsy study of 225 women without overt breast disease showed a 19% incidence of macrocysts, while another study found 27% incidental cysts in 300 breasts removed for cancer[23].

Cysts are frequently asymptomatic; often they are noticed by accident when the woman or a sexual partner touches the breast. A cyst may be symptom free and then suddenly become painful, probably due to irritation from leakage of fluid into nearby tissue. Pain may also occur on disappearance of a cyst, if it ruptures or suddenly empties its contents into a duct. The pain experienced is unrelated to the size of the cyst or to the woman's menstrual cycle. Although usually not symptom producing, cysts are still one of the most common reasons for breast clinic visits, either because of their sudden appearance, or because they have become painful. Cysts located behind the nipple, especially if they enlarge rapidly, may promote nipple retraction, an occurrence that often leads the concerned woman to seek medical consultation. Nipple discharge may occasionally occur if a leaking cyst is in direct communication with the nipple. In this case the discharge would predictably be the brownish (clear tea coloured) fluid typical of cysts.

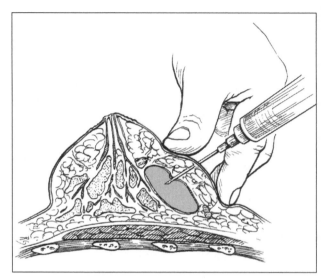

Surgical excision used to be the treatment for all cysts but now surgery is virtually never done unless there is a concern that the cyst may be masking a deeper cancer. They are either left alone or emptied by needle aspiration (see Figure 18).

Figure 18. Technique for aspirating a cyst
(Powell D.E. & Stelling C.B., The Diagnosis and Detection of Breast Disease, C.V. Mosby Co., ©1994)

5. Duct Ectasia

Duct ectasia usually begins as an inflammatory condition of a major duct deep to the nipple and areola, although the exact etiology is unclear. The woman may or may not be aware of the inflammation when it occurs. The theory is that a duct mastitis (perhaps from lactation or diabetes related), a post-surgical infection, or an autoimmune inflammation leads to weakening of the duct's myoepithelial layer and to subsequent dilation and poor clearance of the duct. Accumulation and stagnation of secretions ensues, causing epithelial irritation. This irritation promotes local sensitivity, inflammatory reactions, and perhaps duct wall ulceration[24,25]. Eventually a reactive fibrosis occurs which causes stiffening, torsion, and shortening of the duct, resulting in an inward pull on the nipple. This process probably unfolds over several years. Whitish or yellowish secretions may be discharged from the nipple.

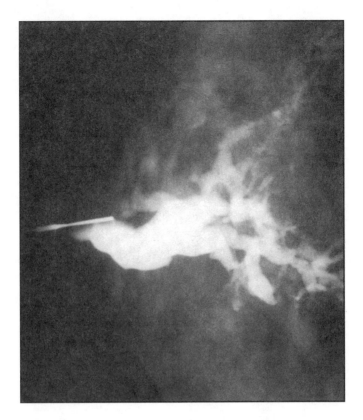

Figure 19. Iodinated contrast image of ectasia of a central breast duct (Powell D.E. & Stelling C.B., The Diagnosis and Detection of Breast Disease, C.V. Mosby Co., ©1994)

Duct ectasia is very common; in a post-mortem study it was found to be present in 25% of women of all ages[26]. It is typically diagnosed in the 40-60 age group, and is believed to be present in 60% of postmenopausal women[27].

While not always symptomatic, duct ectasia usually presents clinically with some or all of the following signs and symptoms:

- nipple retraction
- creamy opaque white/yellow nipple discharge, usually sporadic, possibly with an unpleasant odour
- small inflammatory reactions
- possible presence of small abscesses

- nipple sensitivity, especially to cold and/or pressure
- episodes of precisely located sharp burning pain, usually experienced behind the nipple, although sometimes in the UIQ
- cold exacerbates the pain[28]
- subareolar tenderness on palpation; there may also be palpable small nodules

The massage therapist should note from the above list that cold applications and touch with pressure may exacerbate the sensitivity of the breast. While much of this reaction comes from direct contact with the nipple and areola, and is therefore not likely to occur in response to breast massage, hydrotherapy applications can have generalized effects. Also, the client may not be comfortable putting pressure on the breast by lying prone, necessitating position adaptations.

Duct ectasia is generally not treated medically, unless for abscess or infection.

Other Common Causes of Benign Breast Lumps

Hematoma
- caused by injury or surgery, anticoagulant use, low platelet count
- feels like any hematoma elsewhere in the body

Lipid Cyst
- usually follows trauma
- feels like a well-defined fatty lump

Abscess (more detail in Mastitis section which follows)
- usually secondary to mastitis
- may result from duct ectasia, diabetes, breast trauma/surgery, steroid treatments, chronic inflammatory diseases (e.g. lupus, rheumatoid arthritis), direct silicone and paraffin implants, tuberculosis
- can be idiopathic
- abscesses are usually firm and painful and accompanied by inflammatory changes and edema

Silicone Injections
- often result in diffuse densities with poor border definition[29]
- not commonly used now, but may have been present for many years

Intramammary Lymph Node
- fairly common
- sometimes enlarge enough to be palpable
- rounded/ovoid; feels much like a cyst
- usually found in the UOQ

Prominent Rib
- not a breast lump; however a prominent rib underlying the breast can cause concern until the woman is reassured about what it is
- often associated with ribcage asymmetry

Mastitis

Lactational Mastitis

Mastitis is inflammation of breast tissue. Most cases are related to breastfeeding (lactational mastitis) and are caused by bacterial infection. The infection becomes established when the organism gains access to the breast's duct system. Milk is an ideal culture medium, and in combination with the warmth and increased vascularization of the breast tissue, it provides a hospitable environment for bacterial proliferation.

Lactational mastitis occurs in 1-5%[30,31] of breastfeeding women; there is a 10% likelihood of recurrence in the same woman with future infants. Infection usually develops in the first month of nursing. Other higher risk times include when the baby begins to teethe (around 6 months) and at weaning or other times of marked reduction in nursing frequency.

During lactation small lesions or cracks can form in the nipple and areola. This is especially true at the beginning of breastfeeding when the tissues are unaccustomed to the new usage. Most women are instructed to chafe their nipples and areolae with a textured cloth during pregnancy in order to help strengthen the skin against breakdown when breastfeeding starts. Nonetheless, approximately 35% develop nipple damage in the first 5 days of lactation[32]. When openings in the skin occur, passage of common bacteria from the baby's mouth into the duct system is facilitated. In some cases transmission occurs without a discernable lesion and may be via the ductal openings in the nipples. Maternal fatigue and problems with nursing technique can be contributing factors.

The bacteria involved are common - usually staphylococcus aureus or epidermis, or an ordinary strain of streptococcus. Staphylococcus aureus is the most frequent cause and is often picked up by the baby in the hospital nursery. Staphylococcal infections typically produce one or more focalized lesions, and are usually confined to one breast segment, at least initially. Streptococcal infestations usually involve the entire breast in a more disseminated pattern.

The infected tissue quickly becomes painful and indurated (hardened), with substantial local inflammation and edema. The woman usually also experiences fever and systemic flu-like illness. The baby is generally not sick or has only minor symptoms.

Lactational mastitis is treated by 10 days of antibiotic therapy. Doctors are knowledgeable about which types of antibiotics are not considered harmful to the baby. Despite being painful, continued breastfeeding is strongly recommended to prevent even more congestion and stasis. The breast needs to be completely emptied several times a day, so supplementary pumping may also be advised. Bed rest and breast support are also recommended. The major risk for the mother is abscess formation, which can cause permanent damage to her breast tissue. Adherence to the 10 day antibiotic course and frequent breast emptying significantly decrease the risk of abscess development.

Many women feel an understandable reluctance to take drugs while breastfeeding and may be inclined to try alternatives like massage therapy. Whether the woman is taking antibiotics or not, cold hydrotherapy (see the 'figure 8 wrap' illustration in the Breast Massage During Pregnancy and Breastfeeding section) can be very effective in helping to manage pain and inflammation, and gentle lymphatic drainage can be used to help reduce congestion. However, any on-site massage techniques involving direct pressure are strongly contraindicated until the infection has subsided. A study[33] of 305 women with acute lactational mastitis in the former Soviet Union, 167 of whom were receiving breast massage from medical personnel and/or self massaging, found that direct massage of the affected breast led to damage of inflamed blood vessel walls and thrombophlebitis, as well as to increased distribution of the organism through the glandular system of the breast. Abscess formation was accelerated and larger abscesses formed. In addition, abscesses were more likely to form at distant sites.

Massage therapists should also have an appreciation of the need for good hygiene when giving breast massage to lactating mothers, especially at the high risk times mentioned above. Since the organisms typically involved are common in our environment, thorough hand washing and careful attention to other standard hygienic precautions will help minimize the risk of transmission during massage therapy.

Non-Lactational Mastitis

Mastitis of the non-lactating breast is not as frequent an occurrence, but it does happen. Non-lactational mastitis is often idiopathic, meaning that the cause cannot be determined. What follows is a list of reasonably common known causes:

1. A progression from duct ectasia.

2. A condition called foreign body mastitis, which is a chronic inflammatory response that can follow implantation of foreign material into the breast, especially silicone[34]. The inflammatory reaction may occur quickly following placement and/or later with implant leakage or rupture. This is a non-infective irritation response and is not adversely affected by hydrotherapy or gentle massage, although there may be concerns about the stability of the implant, as will be discussed in a later section.

3. Breast trauma or surgery resulting in an inflammatory reaction, and perhaps infection.

4. Circumstances involving poor immune response, for example diabetes or long-term steroid use.

5. A complication of viral infections like mumps (viral mastitis).

6. Associated with inflammatory autoimmune conditions, for example rheumatoid arthritis or lupus.

7. Communication from a nearby infected structure, e.g. a sebaceous cyst, or resulting from a blood-borne infection from another part of the body.

8. A fairly common complication of tuberculosis and typhoid fever. These conditions, especially TB, can be encountered in North America, or may be seen by the massage therapist working in other countries.

Neither lactational nor non-lactational mastitis is associated with increased cancer risk. There are, however, a few dangerous inflammatory types of breast cancer which can onset quickly with considerable mastitis. For this reason, inflammatory reactions in the breast should always be thoroughly investigated for cause.

Breast Abscesses

An abscess is a localized collection of pus, often encapsulated, which can develop anywhere in the body. Abscesses are frequent sequelae of bacterial mastitis, both lactational and non-lactational. The causes are therefore essentially the same as those given for mastitis in the above section, excepting those with non-bacterial origins. Statistically, 5-10%[35,36] of bacterial infections in the breast lead to abscess. The organism usually involved is staphylococcus aureus, which tends to form localized pockets of infection from the outset.

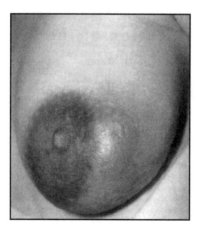 An abscess will typically present as a firm tender lump with local inflammatory changes and edema. A fluctuant centre may be palpable. The woman may also experience fever and general malaise. When an abscess develops during antibiotic use (or just following it), both the local and systemic symptoms may be temporarily masked.

Figure 20. A breast abscess which has progressed to the point that necrosis has begun to develop in the overlying skin. (Hughes L.E., Mansel R.E., Webster D.J.T., Benign Disorders and Diseases of the Breast, Baillière Tindall, ©1998)

Once an abscess has formed, surgery to drain it is indicated. If the woman is breastfeeding she must stop nursing from the affected breast, although frequent pumping is instituted. Antibiotic therapy is begun or continued, and recovery is expected in 2-4 weeks. The recurrence rate for breast abscesses is 9-15%[37].

Massage treatment concerns are similar to those for mastitis. While hydrotherapy and lymph drainage can be very helpful in reducing edema and the discomforts of inflammation, any techniques which could disrupt the abscess, traumatize the tissue, or promote organism spread must be avoided until the doctor indicates that sufficient resolution has been achieved. There is an added concern about hygiene related to the incision site, which often has open tubes for drainage. As well, even if the client is being given a massage without treating the affected breast, the therapist must be cautious when positioning her to avoid stressing the recent surgical site or compromising any drainage tubes. The majority of abscesses are parenchymal or subareolar (see Figure 21), in other words related to

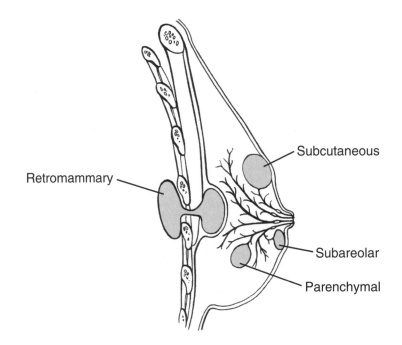

Figure 21. Breast abscess locations

the lobar system, and stem from lactational mastitis. A breast abscess in a woman who does not have duct ectasia, has not had a recent surgery or trauma, and is not breastfeeding, especially if it is found in a more uncommon location, may be indicating an underlying pathology.

Mastalgia - Causes of Breast Pain

Mastalgia is pain experienced in breast tissue. It is a common occurrence - in statistics gathered in Great Britain, mastalgia accounted for approximately half of presentations to breast clinics and the majority of breast related consultations in general practice[38]. Despite this type of statistic, breast pain is very under reported. For example, one British study found that 60-70% of women admitted on direct questioning to experiencing cyclical breast pain but only 3.4% had ever sought treatment[39]. Nonetheless, breast pain can be quite intense and of long duration, adversely affecting quality of life in many cases.

Mastalgia is a symptom; it is not a condition in itself. Of considerable significance to the massage therapist is the fact that 10-13% of breast pain reflects causes outside the breast, usually musculoskeletal[40]. It is also valuable to be aware that pain originating in the breast is often referred to the axilla and upper medial arm.

Over the years various theories have been advanced about what causes or aggravates breast pain. These assumptions have recently been subject to more scientific scrutiny. The results so far seem to indicate that neurosis and generalized water retention, both popular hypotheses, are not involved. Caffeine consumption and reduced levels of essential fatty acids do appear to play a role[41].

Most mastalgia is cyclical, meaning that its pattern corresponds to the menstrual cycle. When it does not, the pain symptom is categorized as non-cyclical.

Cyclical Mastalgia

It is common for women to experience fullness, heaviness, and discomfort in their breasts 3-7 days before the onset of menstruation. The degree of discomfort varies from negligible (heightened awareness) to intense pain. It ceases or greatly diminishes when the menstrual period begins. Discomfort significant enough to be categorized as pain is believed to be an exaggerated version of normally occurring breast tenderness in the luteal phase of the menstrual cycle. Extended versions of the cyclical pattern, called 'prolonged cyclical mastalgia', can start soon after the period ends and gain intensity through to the next one.

The problem in cyclical mastalgia relates to the hormones which on a monthly basis prepare the breast tissue for pregnancy. When mastalgia is present, especially in severe cases, excess estrogen can usually be detected. This estrogen predominance can be relative (insufficiency of counterpart hormones) or absolute[42]. Cyclical mastalgia responds to hormonal manipulation and usually improves when the woman goes on the birth control pill, as long as the dose is not too high in estrogen. It also virtually always ends at menopause, although hormone replacement therapy can prolong cyclical mastalgia and, being estrogen based, often intensifies it.

Another contributing factor is breast nodularity. Nodular tissue areas can become especially tender in conjunction with premenstrual changes in the breast. Fibroadenosis and sclerosing adenosis are most likely to be implicated.

Most cyclical mastalgia is experienced in the upper outer quadrant. It is often bilateral, but unilateral presentations are not uncommon. The mean age of women reporting symptoms of cyclical mastalgia is 34[43].

Non-Cyclical Mastalgia

One of the most frequent causes of non-cyclical mastalgia is breast or nipple pain in breastfeeding mothers, usually as a result of mastitis or problems with lactation. Postural imbalances, prior injuries, or poor positioning during nursing may create or exacerbate musculoskeletal factors and add to the experience of pain.

Non-cyclical mastalgia from other origins is seen in women who are a bit older. The mean age is 43[44]. This statistic reflects the fact that duct ectasia is one of the most frequent causes, and duct ectasia is the most common ANDI condition in women over 40. Most non-cyclical mastalgia is unilateral, although this is by no means exclusively true, and pain levels score lower on average than for cyclical mastalgia.

Another fairly common occurrence is scar tissue in the breast which develops into a long-term pain focus. The scar may originate from an injury, an old abscess site, or a surgical incision. Breasts do not contain usable planes of dissection, so surgical cuts have to be made bluntly through the tissues; this can lead to less compliant, more irritating types of scarring. One source found old biopsy scars to be strongly implicated, comprising 8% of the problems in the non-cyclical pain group studied[45]. Closer investigation revealed that in several of the cases the original procedure had been complicated by infection or hematoma.

Breast implants can also be a source of pain, especially if there is reactive mastitis, capsular contracture, implant leakage which irritates nearby tissue, or calcification.

When the pain source is not actually in the breast, the cause is frequently a cervical spine problem - most typically, disc protrusion in younger women and degenerative changes in older women. In this circumstance the breast pain is part of a more generalized pattern including projection into the axilla, shoulder, and medial arm. Brachial plexus compression syndromes (including cervical rib) are also common and can cause similar pain syndromes involving the breast as well as the chest wall, arm and hand.

Muscular origins are also common. One study reported that 90% of its participants with unilateral non-cyclical breast pain had musculoskeletal causes, and noted that many in their subject group lived in a working class area and had factory jobs with repetitive arm movements. "The breast pain was often diffuse, with marked tenderness over the lateral border of pectoralis major suggesting a pectoral fasciitis[46]."

Myofascial trigger points may also be responsible for a significant amount of pain referral to the breast[47]. The most likely source is pectoralis major. Also fairly common are breast-referring trigger points in the scalenes, especially the anterior scalene, and pectoralis minor. An occasional source is serratus posterior superior.

The breasts may also be a site of pain referral from viscera, particularly the heart and the digestive tract. What follows is a list of the more common visceral origins of non-cyclical mastalgia:

- angina pectoris, heart attack, heart infections, and other causes of heart pain
- cholelithiasis (gall stones)
- esophageal lesions
- hiatus hernia
- pleurisy
- pulmonary tuberculosis

Tietze's Syndrome, also called costochondritis, is a condition which can affect one or more of the costal cartilages deep to the breast. The cartilage becomes painfully enlarged. Pain increases with palpation of the cartilage, with stress of the affected rib(s), and with pressure applied to the overlying breast. This condition is a differential diagnosis for non-cyclical mastalgia and results in pain experienced 'under' the medial aspect of the breast.

Some researchers have also noted that breast pain of psychosomatic origin may occur, especially if the woman has a history of sexual trauma or abuse.

Ominous Signs

An ominous sign or symptom is one which suggests the possibility of a dangerous cause. The term is used universally to denote the possibility of a serious origin for signs and symptoms which are not in themselves diagnostic but warrant deeper investigation. In the breast context, an ominous sign is one that points to the possibility of cancer.

It is essential for the massage therapist to be aware of signs/symptoms which are suggestive of breast cancer and need careful medical examination. It is equally important to understand that none of these findings is in itself a clear indicator of cancer, and in all cases odds are good that the cause is benign. The sensitive practitioner will communicate, along with advice to seek immediate medical evaluation, a balanced view of the greater likelihood of a non-cancer diagnosis.

Breast cancer fear is understandably strong in most women. The massage therapist should not underestimate the negative effect casual, misinformed, or unsettling remarks can have on a client. Two pieces of information can be helpful to know in this respect:

1. The term dysplasia, when used to describe changes in the breast, does not have the same pre-cancerous connotation as it does, for example, in the cervix or colon[48].

2. Ninety percent of cases brought to medical attention are benign[49].

The breast signs and symptoms commonly considered ominous are:

1. **Nipple Discharge:** Spontaneous nipple discharges are always cause for further investigation although in most cases the etiology is benign. Only 5-7% are caused by cancer[50]. When not associated with lactation, most nipple discharge is caused

by duct ectasia, hormone imbalance, the birth control pill, or dopamine antagonist drugs. Milky types are virtually never ominous. A clear brown tea coloured discharge is typically fluid leaking from a cyst near the nipple, or the result of a cyst rupture. The most worrisome are blood or blood-related discharges -15% are cancerous. Also, a colourless watery type, which is more rare, is closely associated with cancer[51].

2. **Nipple Retraction:** Nipple retraction indicates that the nipple is being pulled inward. The most likely causes are normal involutional fibrosis and duct ectasia. Cancers, especially subareolar ones, can cause tissue changes which result in pulling stresses on the nipple. A retracted nipple can be seen in the cancerous breast in Figure 24.

3. **Nature of the Lump:** Differential diagnosis by palpation alone is impossible, and not all cancers have a characteristic palpatory presentation. There are, however, some general statements that can be made about the usual characteristics of an ominous lump:

   • is very hard, sometimes cartilaginous, in quality
   • feels like a discrete mass with well defined borders
   • is not painful (only 6-7% of breast cancers are discovered because of pain, and these are often more progressed)
   • does not change with the monthly hormonal cycle
   • moves poorly in relation to adjacent breast tissue, especially with circular palpation

The last point is an important one which needs elaboration. As is illustrated in Figure 22, lesions which are extensions of the lobar unit in the breast tend to move readily and naturally with the surrounding breast tissue, although this freedom of movement may be compromised by fibrous involutional change. Malignancies, however, do not respect tissue boundaries and grow into neighbouring structures invasively. As the palpator moves the breast, the cancerous lump's incursion into its surrounding tissues creates a lack of pliancy and results in a feeling of 'dragging over' the spot, or of mobilizing a large section of the breast en masse.

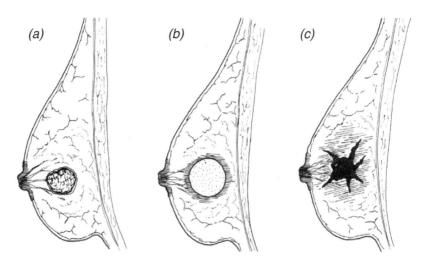

Figure 22. Mobility of breast lumps in relation to surrounding breast tissue: (a) fibradenoma (b) cyst (c) cancer. The shaded area indicates the amount of breast tissue moving with the lump. (Hughes L.E., Mansel R.E., Webster D.J.T., Benign Disorders and Diseases of the Breast, Baillière Tindall, ©1998)

4. **Changes in Breast Contour:** The invasion of cancer into its neighbour tissues changes the interplay of tissue relationships and tensions. As is seen in Figure 23, one of the results can be 'contraction' of the skin surface. Even small dimples or puckers may represent significant cancerous growths below. The change in skin contour is sometimes more easily noticed when the woman bends forward, or when the breast tissue is moving. The most common explanations for this type of skin surface presentation are the presence of a scar or the fibrosity of an old injury site. Any newly developed or unexplained change in skin contour should be closely examined by a doctor.

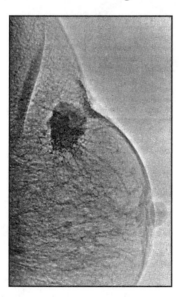

Figure 23. Skin surface 'puckering' caused by an underlying carcinoma (Cawson R.A., McCracken A.S., Marcus P.B., Zaatori G.S. Pathology., The Mechanisms of Disease, 2nd ed., © C.V. Mosby Co, 1998)

5. **Changes in Skin Colour or Texture:** There are numerous reasons for changes in breast skin quality and texture that are not ominous. There is, however, a characteristic one which develops when a breast carcinoma advances into the tiny lymph vessels of the skin and subcutaneous tissues. It is called peau d'orange (Fr: orange peel) because it resembles the surface quality of an orange, and to some extent because it also takes on an amber/orangy colour. Figure 24 shows a progressed cancer which is very illustrative of peau d'orange. It is not common to see a cancer this advanced; however the massage therapist might notice a small patch of characteristically discoloured or textured skin.

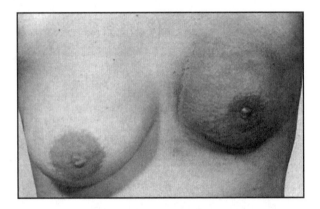

Figure 24. Peau d'orange in advanced breast cancer
(Cawson R.A., McCracken A.S., Marcus P.B., Zaatori G.S., Pathology: The Mechanisms of Disease, 2nd ed., C.V. Mosby Co., ©1998)

6. **Atypical Presentations of Breast Lesions:** As has been mentioned in previous sections, unexplained, atypically located abscesses and postmenopausal cyst activity are two examples of potentially ominous variations of usually non-ominous tissue developments.

7. **Skin Breakdown:** Spontaneous or unexplained skin ulceration, poor healing of a skin injury, or skin breakdown under minimal stress may all be indicators of cancer, although other origins are very possible, for example diabetes and hypersensitivity reactions.

8. **Changed Prominence of Veins:** The practitioner should take note of changes in the prominence of the superficial breast veins, since enlargement may be a sign of the increased metabolic activity of cancer. This finding is also typical of early stage pregnancy, mastitis and breast abscess, and tissue trauma. It is also not uncommon for varicosities to develop at an old injury or surgery site, so vein prominence is not a strongly ominous sign. It can, however, be an important indicator in some cases.

Men Get Breast Conditions Too[52]

Men have a small amount of breast parenchyma and, although it is much more rare, can develop all the benign and malignant conditions women do.

Sources generally agree that there are between 800 and 1000 cases of breast cancer diagnosed in men each year in the United States. The average age of diagnosis in men is 59 (5-10 years higher than the female average). The prognosis is frequently poor because ominous signs are often overlooked and late diagnosis is unfortunately typical. Most male breast cancers are located subareolarly or in the UOQ, although all lumps found in the male chest area should be carefully followed up medically. The most common ominous presentations are: bloody nipple discharge, nipple retraction, nipple or skin ulceration, unexplained tenderness, and lump fixation.

Gynecomastia is the term used to describe breast enlargement in men. There are a number of potential causes. Some degree of gynecomastia is a normal part of male aging, as the predominance of testosterone declines and estrogen becomes relatively more influential. Body type inheritance can also be a factor. Other causes include fatty deposition (considered non-pathological); hormone imbalance (estrogen excess or androgen deficiency); drug side effect (numerous drugs can be implicated, some of which are: valium, steroids, insulin, dilantin, digitalis, several antidepressants, hormone therapies, marijuana); cancers and other disorders of the testicles, adrenals, thyroid, and kidneys; some lung pathologies; cancer and cirrhosis of the liver; granulomatous diseases like tuberculosis.

In addition to gynecomastia, the breast conditions seen most commonly in men are lipoma (benign fatty mass), abscess (diabetes is a frequent underlying cause), and ductal papilloma (benign endothelial tumour). Least common are lobule-originating formations like cysts, since men usually have little or no defined lobular structure.

Breast Implants

It is estimated that between 1 and 2 million women in the United States have breast implants. Approximately 70-80% were placed for cosmetic reasons, and the remaining 20-30% were used in breast reconstruction[53]. The worldwide number is approximately three million[54]. Reconstructions are most commonly done after cancer-related mastectomies, but may also be indicated following traumas and burn injuries and for some breast malformations. The estimated number of women who have had augmentation mammoplasty (breast enlargement) in the U.S. is 0.65-2% of the female population[55]. Adverse publicity in the early 1990's caused a 50% drop in implant procedures, but interest is increasing again, and in 1996 sales of implants equalled 1991 figures.

Massage therapists need to be informed of the basic facts about breast implants, including post-surgical issues and the health and comfort considerations that can arise for massage therapy clients who have implants. While this obviously applies to the practitioner who offers breast massage, there are also some important points of awareness for those who do not. For example, implants can make a client uncomfortable lying in some positions; they may also be sources of non-breast pain. Although there is very little reference material on the efficacy of manual techniques for breasts containing implants, it is our responsibility to consider what is known and what we can safely conclude would be suitable guidelines for the responsible practitioner.

There has been considerable controversy about whether breast implants cause general health problems. As yet there are few definitive answers about the causes and treatment of the systemic symptoms some women develop. A general understanding of the history and the health questions surrounding breast implants helps the massage therapist to be responsive and sensitive to clients who have them.

History

The first reported implant procedure took place in 1895, when a surgeon in Germany used a lipoma from a patient's back to replace breast tissue lost from removal of a benign tumour[56]. The procedure was not successful because the fat was resorbed. Direct implantation, generally of paraffin, silicone, and also of polyvinyl sponges in the 1950's, was the only available procedure from the 1890's until the development of the modern implant. These techniques, where the material was injected or placed directly into the breast tissue, were fraught with high incidences of infection, hard mass formation, calcification, cyst and sinus development, breast malformation, and loss of skin integrity. They also made routine breast monitoring more difficult. Injection of silicone was prohibited by the United States Food & Drug Administration in 1976. It should be noted, however, that direct implantation of both silicone and paraffin has been used more recently than 1976 in other parts of the world, especially Far East countries like Japan and Vietnam. Massage therapists may well encounter clients who have had this type of procedure.

The modern silicone implant has been available since 1962. Its development reflected the need to produce a viable product with a higher standard of safety and patient satisfaction. All implants have a casing, usually called the shell, and are filled with a gel/fluid material. In the earliest implants the shell was made of a thick silicone rubber and the fill substance was quite dense. The surgeon 'tacked' the implant to the woman's connective tissue, generally with Dacron mesh or silicone tabs. This tacking technique was discontinued in the 1970's because it was found to cause increased fibrosity and unnatural fixation of the implant. These early implants were very stable, meaning they contained their fill material well and rarely ruptured, but they had a stiff, artificial look and feel. Manufacturers began to produce implants with thinner shells and less viscous silicone polymer fills. The problem then became seepage of the gel material through the shell. This continues to be an issue with current day implants. Beyond extrusion of fill through a ruptured shell, which is a problem on the more macro level when it occurs, oils routinely release in small amounts from the silicone fill and seep through the elastomer shell fabric. This is referred to as 'gel bleed'.

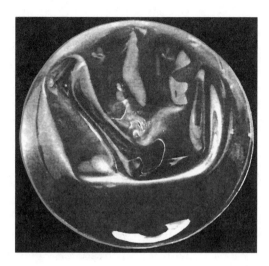

Figure 25. Silicone breast implant

Since the 1980's, shell improvements have helped reduce gel bleed by about 90%, depending on the design. There continues to be a tension, however, between the quest for a natural feeling, cosmetically satisfactory implant and health concerns about fill seepage. Various configurations have been tried, including a double lumen implant with a silicone gel filled centre and a saline filled outer envelope, which was introduced in the hope that it would eliminate silicone bleed. It helps, but has not been completely successful.

Although medical grade silicone is widely believed to be one of the most inert materials in existence, concerns about the safety of silicone gel breast implants resulted in increasing public attention through the 1980's. Case reports describing unexplained symptoms like weakness, chronic fatigue, myalgias and arthralgias, vague generalized upper torso pain, unexplained fever, burning breast pain, rashes, and so on, appeared in medical journals and in the press. In some instances onsets of known rheumatologic diseases were attributed to silicone breast implants.

Despite protest from the medical community and implant manufacturers, the U.S. Food & Drug Administration was unable to overlook the numerous contentions of silicone implant related health problems. In October, 1991 they concluded that while there was no evidence that silicone gel filled implants were unsafe, there was also insufficient evidence to prove safety. On January 6, 1992 a voluntary moratorium was announced. In April of 1992 the FDA clarified the specifics of its position as follows: During the moratorium silicone gel implants would not be available for augmentation, but could be used for reconstruction procedures provided the patient was judged not suitable for saline implants and the use of the silicone products conformed with FDA Internal Review Board protocols. This meant that all women receiving the gel implants would agree to be registered and to participate in a study. The study is known as the Silicone Gel Adjunct Study or the Phase II study.

This study and many others are proceeding with a high degree of participation by researchers, plastic surgeons, and manufacturers. Restrictions on the use of silicone implants were not adopted by all countries; in Great Britain, for example, they have been used freely throughout the past decade. Research conducted in such jurisdictions is being contributed to the overall effort.

The voluminous medical journal literature on the safety of silicone breast implants is fascinating to read, in part because it contains a huge range of opinion, and also because the conflicting elements of self-interested agendas and concerns about public health are both clearly present and often not well resolved. As will be discussed in more detail shortly, the investigation has largely focused on whether the implants can be shown to cause the onset of connective tissue or rheumatologic diseases. In 1995 the FDA Commissioner announced that silicone gel implants do not appear to cause increased incidence of CT disease in users. Manufacturers have been involved in a final phase study in preparation for pre-market approval application. Approval of renewed open access to silicone gel breast implants in the United States seems likely in the not-too-distant future.

Before the moratorium, 80-85% of breast implants used were silicone-filled and most of the rest were saline[57]. Saline implants are available without restriction or control, although in 1995 the FDA announced several studies to test them. They are generally considered safe and have a high patient satisfaction rating[58]. They are not without their problems, however. For one thing, the shells of saline implants are still made of silicone, although of the less contentious silicone elastomer material. They are also filled, or 'inflated', by the surgeon at the time of the procedure, so human error can be a factor. As well, silicone implants have a fairly high spontaneous deflation rate - in one study of 504 subjects, 51 had experienced a deflation[59]. Experimentation with new fill substances, including hydrogels and triglycerides which are considered harmless when absorbed, is underway. Some are already in use in Europe.

The Silicone Controversy

Medical science contends strongly that the medical grade silicone polymers and elastomers used in breast implants and 1000 or more other clinical uses are inert and nonbiodegradable. Although not everyone agrees, it is certainly true that medical use of silicone is widespread and generally not accompanied by the controversy that surrounds breast implants.

Silicone products can be produced in a full array of liquid to solid forms. Some studies suggest that the gel manifestations may evoke an immune response not seen with the more solid forms (for example joint and facial prostheses) because of their tendency to bleed oils. On the other hand, liquid forms of silicone are routinely encountered, apparently safely, by people such as diabetics whose insulin typically contains some silicone. It is possible that breast tissues react differently to gel exposure than bones and blood vessels. It is also true that there are numerous different silicone gel formats; the breast implant formulations may initiate specific immunologic or delayed hypersensitivity reactions. It has also been postulated that leaked silicone oils ingested by macrophages may be converted to silica, or that silica may be released from the implants. Silica is known to generate immunological responses.

Evidence that placement of silicone implants promotes local inflammation and fibrosis reactions is not disputed. Medical grade silicones invoke the standard foreign body response of immune system attack followed by encapsulation. In other words, immune cells first attempt to phagocytose (consume) the material. If this is not possible, the next step is to encase it within host tissue membranes.

The body reacts to a breast implant shell as it would to any foreign material. With or without seepage of silicone products, the body's defences will mount an inflammatory response followed by formation of a fibrous capsule around the implant. The controversy arises about whether there are reactions to breast implants that extend beyond this expected local reaction to a foreign body invader.

Macrophages are immune cells which arrive soon after implantation. Their role, via phagocytosis, is to remove any dead or damaged tissues and to attempt to eliminate the foreign substance. If the offending material is nonbiodegradable, in other words cannot be broken down by the macrophages, they fuse with giant cells to intensify the attack. If the material still cannot be destroyed, the giant cells form layers of connective tissue around it to wall it off. The macrophages persist at the scene - around the implant and within the fibrous capsule - in varying numbers and at various activity levels over time.

Additionally, macrophages play an important role in the activation of inflammatory processes. They do this via their own chemical reactions to antigens and also through alerting T-cells. Macrophages with Class II HLA molecules are involved in activating T-cells in response to foreign materials. They therefore may become implicated in promoting autoimmune or delayed hypersensitivity reactions.

The oils which 'bleed' through the breast implant shell are mostly picked up by macrophages and trapped in the capsule wall, but detection in nearby lymph nodes is relatively common. These oils are hydrophobic, so must travel either by local seepage or inside phagocytotic cells like macrophages. Some sources contend that silicone oils are routinely transported by these cells to distant locations. This contention may be supported by findings that the element silicon can be detected near an implant, and with diminishing concentration in tissues moving away from the breast. Blood silicone levels are also demonstrably higher in women with implants[60].

The question is: Does this information about macrophage activity around the implant and the possible role of immune system cells in picking up and moving silicone products to other locations in the body provide a basis for a possible immune-mediated systemic reaction to silicone breast implants?

Is There a Connective Tissue Disease Connection?

In the 1970's anecdotal reports began to surface describing a relatively small but notable number of cases in which women who had received silicone gel breast implants later claimed to have developed either a recognized rheumatological disease or unexplained symptoms suggestive of an autoimmune disorder.

Onsets of most of the known connective tissue, autoimmune, and rheumatic diseases have since been attributed to breast implants. Examples include polymyositis, fibromyalgia and chronic fatigue syndrome, all of the inflammatory arthritides, Raynaud's Syndrome, neurological conditions like amyotrophic lateral sclerosis (ALS) and multiple sclerosis, and thyroid conditions like Grave's Disease and Hashimoto's thyroiditis. The term 'human adjuvant disease' is often used to represent the relationship that may exist between an implant and symptom development in the host's body. Of all the diseases that might be precipitated by reactions to implants, scleroderma and systemic lupus erythematosus have been considered the most likely candidates; the possibility of a connection to these conditions has been especially closely scrutinized.

To date, close to a million women have been involved in a multitude of small and large scale studies in several countries. These studies have examined possible links between silicone breast implants and virtually all the known CT and rheumatological conditions, as well as numerous other diseases under consideration. No association with any known condition has been reliably demonstrated. The body of research is very convincing. On October 22, 1995, the American College of Rheumatology issued a statement concluding that "...these studies provide compelling evidence that silicone implants expose patients to no demonstrable additional risk for connective tissue or rheumatic disease[61]." There are now several excellent literature reviews[62,63,64] available to the interested reader which help to summarize this body of study results. The findings are described in terms like 'strikingly consistent'.

Interestingly, two studies which reported no evidence of increased rheumatic disease noted that their subject groups with implants reported more rheumatic symptoms[65,66]. Also, one large cohort study of 395,543 health professional women found that their only statistically significant category was 'other CT diseases'[67]. Herein lies the problem. Women are complaining of symptoms strongly suggestive of connective tissue conditions without having any of the known diseases. This is where a great deal of 'spin' enters the picture as the stakeholders in this controversy assume various explanatory postures. Most of the plastic surgery community and the breast implant business interests are declaring themselves vindicated. They assert that women are not getting ill from silicone implants and tend to explain the reported health complaints as an almost inevitable result of the intense media and legal hype that has prevailed in the past 10 years.

Truthfully, mass media coverage of health problems attributed to breast implants, legal case outcomes including large settlements, and speculation about the potential hazards of silicone exposure must be considered possible factors in the generation of illness accounts. The volume of complaints did increase substantially with public exposure to the breast implant controversy. It has also been noted by many medical personnel and researchers that 'silicone anxiety' is strong and not entirely rational in the consumer mindset. Any thoughtful person trying to reach a balanced understanding of the issues would find it difficult to imagine that women with silicone implants could be unaffected by the stories they hear and the fears of debilitating disease that are invoked.

However, it is hard to be completely comfortable dismissing the numerous case reports out of hand. Many of the women in question are very sick. Some doctors, based on their clinical experiences, are urging caution in declaring implants harmless for everyone. One plastic surgeon[68], in a letter to the Medical Journal of Australia, chides an author published in another professional journal for overzealous conclusions about the safety of silicone implants. He points out that many surgeons like himself see a noteworthy number of puzzling incidences of "a less well defined conglomerate of symptoms which could be either an immunological disease or a connective tissue disease". Breast clinic reporting also fairly consistently identifies a small but significant number of women with this profile of mixed CT disease-like symptoms.

'Silicone associated disorder', a new term, has been put forward to describe the systemic reaction that some women appear to be having to silicone implants. Other names, for example 'siliconosis', 'silicone reactive disorder', 'silicone implant associated syndrome', and 'silicone toxicity', have also been put forward. One source predicts that as many as 20% of women with silicone breast implants will develop symptoms somewhere on the mild-moderate-severe scale[69]. The majority of reported cases involve an idiosyncratic cluster of musculoskeletal complaints. The clinical presentation most closely resembles that of fibromyalgia. It is possible that what is being described is an immune-mediated reaction rather than a specific immune or autoimmune condition. It is also possible that a new disease state has been created or identified.

Even in the more resistant quarters of the pro-silicone camp many concede that if a connection does exist it probably involves activation of a genetic predisposition in a certain percentage of women. Although there are identified genetic markers for many of the known diseases, there is no general test for CT condition predisposition. There are also no specific or definitive tests for silicone body content or body reactions to silicone. Because it is believed so strongly to be inert, no test or marker has been developed to investigate for silicone antigenic reactions.

One interesting study[70] involved 199 subjects, of whom 77 were symptomatic women with implants and others were asymptomatic women with implants, healthy controls without implants, and symptomatic fibromyalgia patients without implants. The symptomatic-with-implants group had to meet the following criteria: systemic symptomatology of >4 months duration which had to be debilitating enough to interfere with activities of daily living, especially work, and not diagnostic of any known rheumatic condition. The researchers set out to determine whether women who developed this type of symptom picture after silicone breast implantation demonstrated any HLA typing patterns.

Human Leukocyte Antigens (HLA's) are inherited cell characteristics whose main purpose is to regulate immune responses to self and non-self antigens. A small percentage of HLA's are implicated in autoimmune diseases. Class II HLA's - the DR, DP, and DQ types - are involved in the regulation of interactions among immune cells like macrophages, B-cells, and T-cells. They are considered important factors in the development of immunologic disorders, and characteristic patterns have been identified. For example, HLA-DR4 is linked with rheumatoid arthritis, -DR2 and -DR3 with lupus, and -DR3 and -DR5 with scleroderma. Interestingly, breast tissue contains more DR+ cells than do tissues in other sites of frequent silicone device implantation.

The study found that women with implants who had developed the symptom profile described above showed statistically significant correlations with HLA-DR53, HLA-DR57, and HLA-DQ2. This is a new pattern not linked to other known rheumatic diseases. The symptomatic subjects were closest in HLA characteristics to the fibromyalgia-without-implants group.

Additionally, 42% of the symptomatic implanted women formed antibodies to their own B-cells, a finding much higher than for the other subject groups (19% of the fibromyalgia patients, 14% of the asymptomatic implant group, and 2% of the healthy controls). Of the symptomatic subjects who produced antibodies to their own B-cells, 81% were HLA-DR53+, compared to 33% of the fibromyalgia group. There was no other significant difference between the symptomatic and asymptomatic implant groups in incidence of the common breast implant related concerns like capsular contracture, lymphadenopathy, or frequency of implant rupture. This research suggests that symptomatic patients with implants may share important genetic characteristics. The researchers propose further investigation of the potential use of HLA-DR53 in particular as a marker to identify women who should perhaps avoid implant use.

In the above study, symptoms appeared on average 9 years after implantation. Several other references also describe an 8-10 year time frame between implantation and systemic symptom development. It is noteworthy that this corresponds with the typical time frame for breakdown of implants, as will be discussed in the next section. In the symptomatic group there was a 47% correlation between implant rupture and formation of autoantibodies. This correlation was not present in the asymptomatic group.

Other research may be pointing to formation of anticollagen antibodies in women with breast implants[71]. Lipid abnormalities have also been noted[72].

Another study[73] looked at responses of monocytes (another type of immune system cell) to a variety of connective tissue proteins, materials common to silicone breast implants, and control substances. The purpose was to see if evidence of developed self-immune reactions could be observed in women with silicone breast implants as compared to non-implanted controls. Subjects who had had implants removed were also included in the study. The results showed that the implant subjects had significantly higher mononuclear cell reactivity to collagen I, collagen III, fibrinogen, and fibronectin than the control group. The strongest immune reaction was against collagen I fibres; the strongest development of self-antigen reaction was against collagen III. In total, 50% of the implanted women showed reactions against one of the above four connective tissue materials, as opposed to the control group at 8%. Thirty-nine percent of the implant group responded to more than one of the antigens; no one in the control group did. With respect to production of antibodies (humoral immunity reactions), 19% versus 4% tested positive. All other tested substances evoked response rates in the two groups that showed no significant differences. There was also no significant difference in reactivity between explanted and still implanted subjects, although the typical period since implant removal was relatively short (mean 13 months).

All of this research is controversial. For example, other studies looking into autoantibody formation in women with breast implants show both positive and negative results[74]. There is much more work to be done in the effort to find tests and/or genetic markers to predict which women are at higher risk.

Other General Health Concerns About Breast Implants

Do Implants Promote Cancer? [75,76,77,78]

Numerous studies, now covering a 10-20 year period, show no evidence of breast implants being implicated in subsequent development of breast cancer. In fact, women with silicone implants may have a slightly decreased incidence of breast cancer compared to matches in the general population. Similar results have been obtained from animal studies. Some research indicates that blood from implanted women may kill cancers in tissue dishes. There is also some evidence that having silicone breast implants may reduce the incidence of non-breast cancers.

A major concern has been whether the presence of implants impedes detection of breast cancers. This has not been found to be true, based on considerable investigation. It is the case, however, that specific additional mammogram views must be taken to ensure thorough evaluation of the implanted breast. Women with implants should make certain that technicians testing them are properly trained to work with their breasts.

There is also no evidence of increased risk of recurrence of cancer in post-mastectomy reconstruction patients, nor any evidence that implants cause delay in diagnosing recurrences, assuming proper mammography techniques are utilized.

Do Implants Cause Problems with Pregnancy, Lactation, or Health of the Child?

Difficulties with lactation may occur. The problem is usually insufficient milk production. Scar tissue may also create obstacles to movement of milk from the breast through the nipple. This is most likely to arise from periareolar inserts of saline implants (the implant shell is inserted through an incision on the edge of the areola and inflated once in position in the breast). This problem can also occur in women with periareolar incisions for other breast procedures.

There is no evidence of silicone related fetal abnormality in animal studies[79]. There are also few anecdotal case reports causing concern in this regard.

One controversial study[80] reported finding "scleroderma-like esophageal dysmotility" in children breastfed by mothers with silicone implants. The children (all symptomatic at the time of the study) were between the ages of 6 months and 16 years. None was currently being breastfed.

Women who want to have breast implants and later breastfeed need to take steps to satisfy themselves that they are comfortable in their understanding of the potential risks and problems.

Common Clinical Problems

While the controversy about whether silicone breast implants promote systemic disease continues to generate collegial debate and interesting research, there are more common clinical issues that arise, most of them local to the implant. Although the majority of women do not have problems with their implants, localized symptoms are common enough that they will undoubtedly be part of the clinical experience of massage therapists who do breast massage.

Post-Surgical Issues

Post-surgical complications fall into the standard categories, most typically infection around the implant and hematoma development. Both cause concern, for the usual reasons, and because they have been found to promote contracture of the fibrous capsule that forms around the prosthesis. Wound dehiscence (bursting open of the wound) can also occur.

From the massage practitioner's point of view, treatment planning should include standard post-surgical guidelines about hygienic precautions and avoidance of overly early on-site work. The immediate goals of massage therapy are to reduce inflammation and pain, to safely optimize circulation and drainage around the surgical site, and to promote overall relaxation. Subsequently, the massage therapist can also help restore good shoulder range of motion, since this may be a problem, especially for women having post-mastectomy reconstruction.

Some surgeons advocate that their patients self massage regularly in the first months following implantation, beginning as soon as they can tolerate it, in order to promote softer capsule formation. This practice will be discussed in more detail shortly. However, in the absence of guidance from research, it makes sense to exercise caution in applying rigorous local massage therapy in the first weeks of the healing process, since this type of stimulation may promote formation of an added volume of protective collagen in the breast.

Capsule Contracture

As has already been discussed, placement of an implant (of any type) activates immune system responses which culminate in the development of a fibrous capsule to surround it. Encapsulation is a normal reaction to foreign material and is to be anticipated whenever such materials are introduced into the body. The capsule begins as loose membrane in the first few months, but by six months post implantation it has become a layer of fibroblasts surrounded by a predominantly avascular acellular collagen sheath. This type of collagen structure can be quite stiff. As well, the transition from loose membrane to collagen capsule involves a reduction in fluid volume that can result in the structure being 'stretched' over the implant. It also tends to undergo a pseudo-contractile process common to scar/capsule formations of this type. The resulting firmness or hardness of the capsule can produce pain characterized by a tight, pressured, or 'drawing' quality that in severe cases may be very intense. It can also promote displacement of the implant and distortion of the breast contour.

The degree of capsule formation and capsular stiffening, or contracture, varies from woman to woman. There may be genetic factors involved. Subclinical infection around the prosthesis (staphylococcus epidermis has been implicated) may play a role. Some doctors advocate inserting antibiotics and steroids around the implant; their effectiveness in producing better capsule results is uncertain.

Capsular contracture is the most common complication of breast implants. The Baker Scale (Classes I to IV) is used to designate degree of contracture. A Class I capsular contracture is pliable and virtually undetectable; a Class IV is hardened to the degree that it is likely to be chronically painful and create breast tissue distortions.

Capsular contracture is regarded as an implant complication when the degree of firmness causes patient dissatisfaction - usually a Class III or IV. Because it frequently generates physical and emotional distress in implanted women, prevention of capsular contracture has received a great deal of attention. Polyurethane foam shells, introduced in the 1970's and strongly advocated by many surgeons throughout the 1980's, were found to promote softer capsules. However, they became implicated in the health controversy surrounding implants and were voluntarily removed from the market by the manufacturer in 1991. Implants with textured surfaces are gaining popularity because they appear to help lessen the formation of higher Baker scale contractures. In post-mastectomy reconstruction, prior use of a tissue expander (explained in the Post-Surgical Breast Massage section) has also been found to reduce poor contracture results. Laser endoscopy is a new technique which looks promising for use in reducing contractures.

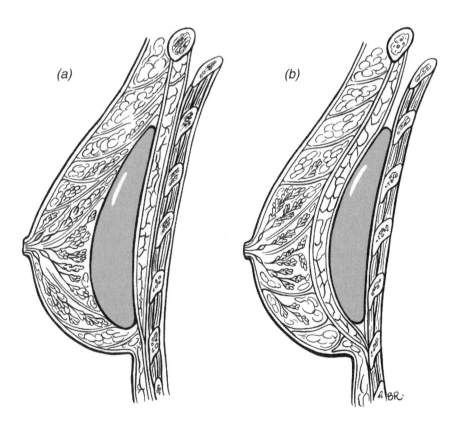

Figure 26. Breast implant placement: (a) subglandular, and (b) submuscular

It has also been found[81] that placement of the implant deep to pectoralis major, usually called submuscular placement, instead of the customary subglandular position on top of the muscle, has a positive effect in reducing the number of Class III and IV capsular contractures formed. See Figure 26 for an illustration of these two implant positions.

Submuscular placement involves creating a fairly large cavity for the implant by dissecting deep to pectoralis major, the superior portion of the external oblique, and some of the serratus anterior digitations. This positioning is believed to help reduce capsular stiffness because of the continuous movement pressures on the implant[82] - several writers refer to this as pectoralis major 'massaging the implant'.

Self massage is recommended by some surgeons to help achieve a softer more pliable capsule. Massage was highly recommended in a 1976 paper on prevention and treatment of fibrous capsules[83]. Interestingly, one surgeon[84] comments: "Constant massage of the breasts, even if it did work, is unnatural. Most patients soon desist." Fortunately this does not appear to be a general sentiment! At the same time, there is little evidence that massage is particularly efficacious in preventing or softening capsular contractures. In fact, overly vigorous massage would probably have the opposite effect. In the case of submuscular placement, however, massage may help reduce spasming in order to optimize the influence of pectoralis major activity on the implant. One source, a surgeon who routinely uses this procedure[85], advocates massage for 15 minutes 3 times a day for the first six months following submuscular implantation.

'Closed capsulotomy' is a procedure which involves tightly squeezing a firm implant in order to disrupt its fibrous envelope and hopefully produce a softer result. It has been seen as a useful procedure because when it works it is instantaneously effective and only momentarily painful. It is most likely to be effective with subglandular placements. In the 1970's and 1980's doctors used closed capsulotomy regularly, and the women themselves (or their partners) were encouraged to do so as well if the capsule began to stiffen. Its use has been associated with a high risk of implant rupture, however, especially with the more thin types of shells. The capsular contracture recurrence rate is also high. The use of closed capsulotomy is now no longer recommended, and if this procedure has been used, the implant manufacturers void the warranty. It is still advocated by some doctors, though, so it may be encountered as a practice used or experienced by some massage therapy clients. Clearly it is not a technique available to the massage practitioner. Massage therapy can be utilized to maximize circulation and drainage and help reduce pain, but aggressive techniques directly addressing the fibrous capsule are more likely to cause problems than solve them.

Massage practitioners should be aware that clients with Class III or IV Baker's contractures are often unable to comfortably lie prone. The stiffest capsules, especially as they age, are also the most likely to rupture or tear under stress. This can influence exercise recommendation in that exercises involving high impact activities like running can be uncomfortable, perhaps even destabilizing for an implant, and contact sports are ill-advised.

Implant Rupture

The old thick-walled shells of the 1960's virtually never ruptured. Some women still have them today. However, rupture is typical of the current thinner-shelled types, whose breakdown over time is considered inevitable. Study reports of current implant rupture rates are fairly consistent; four examples are listed below:

1. Case review of 749 women; 43 experienced implant ruptures in the first 5 years[86]

2. 70% of implants rupture between 6-15 years; 100% likelihood that an implant will rupture at some point after it passes the 10 year mark[87]

3. Failure rate of over 50% beginning at 7-8 years, increasing progressively[88]

4. Rupture frequency correlates with implant age; loss of implant strength and integrity closely correlates with >10 years of age[89]

Although trauma to the implant can cause tearing/rupture, most ruptures do not have a traumatic cause. As the shell ages it becomes increasingly susceptible to loss of surface integrity. The reason is not well understood - lipid infiltration of the elastomer shell is a theory that has gained some acceptance.

A rupture may or may not be painful at the time. If there is pain, it is usually felt as a persistent local burning sensation. Visible or palpable alteration in the shape or texture of the implant may occur. Gel from a ruptured implant can also be mobilized into nearby tissues, and has been found in locations such as the chest wall, axilla, down the arm, in lymph nodes, and occasionally in the abdomen and the pleural space. Pain can occur in these locations, and 'masses' of gel may be observed. Brachial plexus compression from silicone has occasionally been reported, as has nipple discharge of implant fill.

Leakage from a torn implant is generally entrapped in a new connective tissue membrane within 2-6 weeks. It is continuously invaded by cicatricial septa which sub-divide the gel into multiple encased droplets in a granuloma type of formation[90].

The massage therapist must be mindful of the risk of tearing an implant with overly firm or 'pointy' direct techniques, or with manipulations which might strongly pull on or stretch the prosthesis and its capsule. Caution about overstressing an implant should increase as it moves beyond six years of age.

Local massage would be contraindicated in the first six weeks following an untreated rupture, and any previously ruptured implant still in place must be approached with caution, both in terms of breast massage techniques and client positioning.

One source[91] states succinctly that women contemplating breast implantation must be made aware of the anticipated 8-10 year obsolescence rate and the likelihood that implant rupture will make removal/replacement necessary.

Calcification[92]

The incidence of calcification is nothing like the 70-75% it used to be with the previous practices of using liquid paraffin and silicone injections, but it does still occur with a smaller percentage of the modern type of breast implant. The exact cause is not known. Calcification is clinically important because it can be quite painful.

One study found that 16% of 150 removed implants had extensive calcification. All had presented as bilateral Baker Class IV contractures, with pain as the chief complaint. Three women had twenty-five year old Dacron backed shells which were still intact but extensively calcified. The remaining implants were 'younger' but had in almost all cases ruptured. None of the implants in place for ten years or less had calcified.

The calcification typically takes the form of white plaque deposits at the capsule-prosthesis interface. It occurs with both silicone gel and saline implants. Less commonly, calcification can be found within the fibrous capsule as zinc-calcium phosphate, a salt which has never been reported in any other human body situation and may be related to the glue sealant used in the manufacture of the shells.

The presence of calcification does not pose any additional concerns for the massage therapist. It is important to be aware that the implant in question is likely to be more than 10 years old and unstable. The client may be restricted by pain from lying in prone or sidelying positions, and may find certain movements and exercises uncomfortable, depending on the exact location of the calcium deposits.

Pain

Pain requiring a few days of medication is expected after most surgical procedures. Women who have had breast surgery frequently experience significant levels of post-surgical pain. This subject will be discussed in a later section. Placement of breast implants is associated with higher frequency and intensity of post-surgical pain than breast surgeries not involving implantation. It is also true that chronic pain following breast implant procedures is fairly common.

One study[93] sent questionnaires to 479 women who had had breast surgeries over a five year period in the following categories: cosmetic augmentation, reduction, mastectomy, and mastectomy with reconstruction (some using implants, others using the woman's own tissues). Fifty-nine per cent (282) responded. Most of the women in all groups reported experiencing intermittent pain. The percentage needing pain medication was: mastectomy 28%, mastectomy plus reconstruction 29%, augmentation 20%, and reduction 9%. It was also noted that peak pain intensity was significantly higher in the augmentation group than the other groups. Interestingly, saline implants were associated with a higher pain response than silicone (33% versus 22%).

The incidence of pain occurring at least one year post surgery was as follows: mastectomy 39%, mastectomy plus reconstruction 49%, augmentation 38%, reduction 22%. In the mastectomy plus reconstruction category, 53% of subjects with implants reported pain lasting beyond one year, in contrast with self-tissue reconstruction subjects at 30%. These surprisingly high numbers once again suggest the need to be mindful that breast pain is often unreported by female clients in massage therapy clinical practices.

Submuscular placement of implants scored 50%, compared to 21% of women with subglandular implants reporting pain after one year. The immediate cause of pain with submuscular implantation is often pectoralis major spasm, which massage therapists can help ameliorate. More long term pain may be due to nerve injury or compression.

Women who have received implants and have an onset of pain after one year are likely developing capsular contracture problems. Incidence was reported in the above study at 8% of mastectomy plus reconstruction subjects (immediate versus delayed reconstruction and prior use of tissue expanders were seen to reduce painful complications) and 30% of augmentation subjects.

Most implant related pain is felt in the breast. It ranges from the pressure/pain characteristic of contracture, to the burning feeling associated with rupture (and sometimes with adverse local immune reactions), to the sharp ache that can be caused by calcification. Women who have had radiation therapy sometimes have more implant related pain, presumably because of tissue changes caused by the radiation. Nerve injury or compression may also cause pain of extended duration. A common example is nipple pain following subareolar entry to place the implant.

It is important for the massage practitioner to be aware, however, that implant generated pain may be felt in other locations. The reader may want to review the Mastalgia section presented earlier for breast referral patterns. Most implant related non-breast pain is felt in the arm and/or axilla, and is usually caused by damage or compression of specific nerves, or perhaps of the brachial plexus. Statistically, women who have had mastectomy reconstructions are more likely to experience pain down the arm than those who have had augmentation[94].

Ischemic pain may develop in the breast or any of the other locations mentioned. It reflects a reduction in blood supply to the tender tissue or to its innervating nerves. The causes include a number of factors, many of which the massage therapist can be highly effective in treating, for example: poor quality scarring, muscle spasm, reduced range of motion in the shoulder, and edema. Other causes include migration of the implant and effects of capsular contracture, which it is not in the massage therapy scope of practice to attempt to correct.

Movement limitations, or alternatively, specific movements which stress or compress the implant capsule, innervating nerves, or neighbouring tissues, can also be a source of pain. Where this type of pain is caused or enhanced by muscular and soft tissue restrictions in the arm, shoulder, or neck, massage therapy can be very helpful.

Submuscular implant placement can give rise to a specific type of pain in the subscapular area and lateral breast, sometimes with observable changes in the lateral breast contour. This pain pattern is likely signalling a problem with the serratus anterior digitations involved in the surgical positioning of the implant. This finding should cause the massage therapist to avoid ipsilateral breast massage until the client has been checked by her surgeon, since it usually means that one or more of the digitations has ruptured or is close to doing so[95].

Another important point of awareness for the massage practitioner is the fact that many women who have had breast surgeries, especially related to implant placement and cancer treatment, experience sensory abnormalities. These often take the form of lost or reduced sensation, but can also manifest as painful experiences like dysesthesia (painful parasthesia) and allodynia (stimuli like pressure and temperature are unexpectedly causing pain).

Removal of the Implant

The majority of women have little or no problem with their implants, once the expected post-surgical symptoms cease, until shell breakdown leads to decision-making about removal and replacement of the aging implant. The remainder will experience ongoing local complications, and a smaller group will develop systemic symptoms of varying degrees of severity. Some women, even without current symptoms, worry about the health concerns that have become associated with silicone implants and question the wisdom of keeping their prostheses in place.

Removal of the implants is not surgically difficult unless there is extensive scar and capsule formation. However, the outcome results of explantation can be confusing to interpret. Reported findings about the efficacy of implant removal for eliminating symptoms range from no change, to definite improvement, to temporary amelioration only. One study showed that women experience increased psychological distress in the year following removal, whether the implants were replaced or not[96]. Another[97] reported that its subjects felt marked relief and anxiety reduction with autologous tissue replacement of their implants, regardless of how much symptom improvement they achieved. This is another subject area where agendas and fixed points of view from all sides may be tainting the results picture.

In one interesting study[98], 37 patients with localized implant failure problems and systemic symptoms "for which no diagnosis could be provided" had procedures to replace their implants with their own tissues (myocutaneous flaps). 'Implant anxiety' and the systemic symptoms were their biggest motivators for seeking the operation. Almost all experienced relief of their systemic symptoms in the immediate term (89%), but the improvement rate fell to 32% after six months. The study concluded that implant removal did not predict success in relieving systemic complaints. The local symptoms, however, which were primarily tightness, achy/throbbing pain, and burning pain, were resolved as a result of the procedure, leading the researchers to conclude that capsular contracture and implant extrusion are probably good indicators for removal of the implants and replacement with autologous tissue.

What is Your Reaction To These Statements?

"Breast massage is like an undetonated bomb that has been neglected on the ethical battlefield of massage therapy in the United States. Until it explodes, most of us are quite comfortable ignoring it. If asked our opinions on the subject, most of us agree that it is indeed a perplexing issue, one deserving both discourse and clarification. But most of us don't do it."[99]

"I believe it is unwise for the massage therapy profession to pose the question of whether or not breast massage is 'appropriate' in an absolute sense. What is really behind this formulation is a societal uncertainty about whether breasts can ever be touched in a non-sexual manner. By 'banning' breast massage, massage therapists as health professionals would be legitimizing this idea and placing its importance above any consideration of a client's health care needs. More subtle, but also significant, is the implication that massage therapists are untrustworthy as a group in a way that doctors, nurses, and X-ray technicians are not."[100]

"Our freedom as individuals stems from being able to make choices. If as consumers we are unaware of all options for maintaining our health - including such treatments as breast massage - we cannot take full charge of our wellbeing."[101]

"The way it currently stands, if a female client seeks breast massage for therapeutic reasons, she is likely to encounter a therapist who feels unclear about, and threatened by, the issue. Since this circumstance is not one that well reflects our capability and professionalism, a resolution to the dilemma of female breast massage is essential."[102]

ISSUES, DECISION-MAKING, AND GUIDELINES FOR THE MASSAGE THERAPIST

Introduction

Most massage therapists are uncomfortable with breast massage. There are many reasons for this discomfort, some of which are personal, some attributable to lack of training, and others which reflect understandable fears about repercussions to themselves or to the massage profession. When asked about their concerns, most massage therapists respond in one or more of the following ways:

- I didn't learn it in school/skipped the class/observed a demo but we didn't do any hands-on work/had one class on it during which I never really got comfortable.

- As a male therapist I feel too vulnerable about the possibility of being accused of abuse or misconduct.

- I guess I'm not very comfortable about breasts, including my own. To me breasts are private... I've never really thought much about breast massage. I hope nobody asks me, and so far no one has.

- The massage profession is trying so hard to overcome associations with the sex trade. We are just newly on the path to professional acceptance, and I think we should be cautious about things like breast massage.

- I wouldn't know what to do or say if I found a lump.

- I've never seen some of these scars and I'm uncertain about working with women who have breast cancer. I think I'd feel totally inadequate.

- I wish I could say I feel more comfortable than I do. I should probably take a workshop or something.

- I probably shouldn't say this, but I'm worried that one of us will get turned on and the situation won't get handled well.

- Three women close to me - my mother, my sister, and a good friend - have died of breast cancer. I know what they went through and I live in fear that it will happen to me. In my head I know breast massage is important. My sister had a good massage therapist and she got a lot of massage, especially after her surgeries. I just get too emotional about breast cancer. I can't get enough professional distance.

- I worry that some women may be re-traumatized by breast massage. Sometimes people with an abuse background agree to things when they aren't really comfortable, or don't speak up when they need to stop. I don't want to be part of anything that might hurt someone.

- When I first graduated I was pretty fervent about the importance of breast massage - I guess I was a bit on the politically correct side. I lost a few clients who just didn't come back when I told them they should have breast massage. They're getting massaged by the competition now.

- There are people in massage school and out in the profession who should not be doing breast massage. Perhaps it's best to leave the issue alone.

- How do you tell if the client is trustworthy and wants breast massage for the right reasons? Or, what about clients who may have an abuse history and don't know it?

- I do give breast massage occasionally when a client asks for it, but I'm not very good at it. I don't really know what I'm doing and I don't like feeling that way.

It is very important not to gloss over or undermine the importance of each of these concerns. Breast massage is complex, not technically, but personally and ethically. It requires the therapist to have a high level of professionalism, self awareness, and interpersonal skill, yet it is probably one of the most poorly trained areas in massage therapy education. And there are risks involved, serious potential implications for both the client and the massage therapist, if the situation goes badly.

So what is the massage therapy profession to do? The surface equanimity that exists at the moment is largely the result of not really facing the issues and not having been pushed to.

Breast health is a vital concern for our clients and an important issue in health care. Women are in need, not only of breast treatment for various legitimate reasons, but of help in becoming more comfortable and confident about breast health care. Some women will not touch their own breasts; many do not do regular breast self examination; most women cannot conceive of how to begin to seek out the breast health services they need. Deep-seated reticence from many causes leads women to avoid routine breast screening and to tolerate pain and physical symptoms that would respond well to treatment. These same elements also ensure that most of our clients do not ask for breast massage, but is that really okay? Massage therapists have an effective set of treatment options to offer and we are holding back.

On the other hand, this is a litigious world, and as a society we do not deal with sexual conduct issues well. These issues are so hot these days that despite the obvious need to contain sexual predators, unresolved dilemmas about proper process, treatment versus punishment, the fairness of 'the rules' and whether they are applied equitably, etcetera, leave most of us with misgivings about the environment in which sexual conduct problems are identified and judged. Taking risks in this arena is something to think twice about. We tend to believe (or fear) that it is possible for an innocent person, or perhaps a slightly misguided but not really harmful person, to get caught up in a whirlwind of sexual misconduct accusations that could potentially ruin his or her reputation and career.

Most of us have not had the benefit of being raised in a family or a culture in which sexual matters are handled in a mature, balanced fashion. It can be difficult to feel confident in one's understanding of what is right, or healthy. This is especially true since massage therapy has an intimate, sensual quality which takes us closer than most professions to the border of what might be considered unacceptable. In our societal context, there is no certainty about whether breasts can be touched without sexual intent or ramification. Breasts are generally not viewed as tissues having ordinary problems and requirements; or alternatively they are seen as just fatty tissue for which massage offers no benefits. It is therefore not a big leap to conclude that breast massage is a non-issue, and to feel comfortable contending that it isn't 'worth it' for the therapist. Even those who clearly perceive that breast health is not a sexual matter can argue that it is safest not to push the issue with breast massage.

For many massage therapists it is uncomfortable even to talk about breast massage with clients. Our own learned uneasiness gets in the way. Trying to be careful and calm while communicating about a subject that we can find hard to talk about matter-of-factly often results in feelings of inadequacy and vulnerability.

As well, the massage therapy profession is still working hard to rid itself of associations with the sexual services industry. Our profession is 'young' and needs to proceed steadily and carefully in directions which will lead to the achievement of full professional status and respectability. The concerns about jeopardizing that effort are very real and important.

The problem with these considerations and apprehensions, despite the many ways in which they are valid and legitimate, is that our profession appears to be overly comfortable with the assumption that they can be taken care of through avoiding breast massage.

Consider the other points of view. Is it conceivable that the health care world will continue to underestimate massage therapy if our profession does not 'step up to the plate' in key areas like breast treatment, despite the challenges? If we restrict demonstration of our professionalism, quality of care, and treatment efficacy to our present safety zones, will we grow as a profession? Is it not possible that massage therapy will lose credibility and respect as women become more knowledgeable and confident about breast care and find that massage therapists are unable to meet their needs?

Is our reluctance about breast massage symbolic of avoidance of a larger responsibility, which is to better understand and define massage therapy's particular blend of physical, psychoemotional, and sociopolitical impacts? What if we are not making distinctions between our personal comfort issues and what is good for the profession? Do we comprehend the scope of what we do and ensure that massage therapists are adequately trained to handle the effects of massage therapy in the non-physical realms? Are we sacrificing breast massage rather than addressing it as an example of how massage treatment focuses complexities in the relationship between body tissues and the human beings they belong to?

Also, is it perhaps a naive assumption that avoiding breast treatment, and by extension breast massage training, will work as a measure to prevent sexual misconduct? Will we achieve better control over the small number of sexual deviants in our midst by not giving them breast massage education? Will implications of sexual service or misunderstandings about massage therapy be taken care of if we ignore the responsibility to clarify what does and does not constitute legitimate treatment in the grayer areas, of which breast massage is just one example? Are the concerns related to working with clients who have abuse histories, including the potential for re-traumatization, limited to their breasts?

These questions have no quick or simple answers. We need to address them, however. Massage therapy is encountering many interesting challenges as it evolves as a profession. Some of these challenges are unique to us and some are shared by others in the health care field. How we handle the issues surrounding breast massage may actually be an important indicator of how ready we are to take our place in the professional realm.

Dianne Polseno Crawford, in a recent article[103] in Massage Therapy Journal, reports on the results of her informal survey of massage therapists and massage therapy schools. They answered questions about their use of and attitudes toward breast massage.

Responses were gathered from 20 schools and 216 therapists. Here are some of the results:

Only 64 of the therapists had received breast massage training

150 considered breast massage therapeutic; 14 said no; 52 were unsure

18 did breast massage regularly

52 would do breast massage if asked; 86 would not; 32 would do it under certain conditions; 38 would refer to another massage therapist; 10 would teach the woman breast self massage

2 of the schools included techniques for treating breast tissue in their program

198 respondents believed we need professional guidelines for breast massage

One of her conclusions, based on reactions to this survey and other related discussions, is that massage therapists tend to view breast massage from an ethical standpoint rather than a therapeutic one. Despite a sense that there is a therapeutic basis for breast massage, seemingly shared by most practitioners, the potential therapeutic value of breast massage therapy is not explored or used as an argument for good training, public education, or research. Much more research is needed into all aspects of massage therapy practice, but in light of the concerns it raises, breast massage research would be especially helpful to establish whether beneficial effects of this treatment justify its use.

Since breast massage is not a well researched area, opinions about its efficacy derive from applying general knowledge about massage effects to the specific nature of breast tissue, and from the clinical successes many of us have had. Despite its low utilization, many clients and therapists are strong advocates of breast massage because of positive results they have experienced.

Breast tissue health is heavily dependent on circulation and drainage. While this is true of tissues in general, there are many reasons why the breast may be particularly vulnerable to chronically reduced blood and lymph flow. Common practices like the wearing of tight breast undergarments are probable contributors to poor breast circulation and clearance. The habitual postures adopted by many women to reduce attention to their breasts promote circulatory and lymphatic congestion. Implants and surgical scarring frequently obstruct drainage channels, and may also result in chronic pain syndromes leading women to adopt protective holding postures.

The types of movement which mobilize breast tissue, and thereby promote blood and lymph circulation, must be created in the absence of inherent musculature. The breasts must either move with the active body or be passively mobilized. Unfortunately, most of the types of exercise which produce breast movement are uncomfortable without tight supportive clothing. While self massage can be a viable alternative, it is not commonly used.

Several years ago I learned of a local oncologist who recommends that all women use rebounders (mini trampolines) on the grounds that they provide the right bouncing action for breast lymph drainage. Because the landing is soft, the exercise can usually be well tolerated without a bra. This story made me think about the breast massage I was doing. I realized I needed to start using techniques which incorporated more 'lift and jiggle', rather than the predominantly circular petrissage of the breast surface that I was accustomed to. My later studies of the anatomy of breast tissue drainage channels supported and reinforced this idea.

On a more subtle level, women frequently feel dissatisfied with, alienated from, or anxious about their breasts. The result can be a lack of ordinary comfort with having them touched or exposed for non-sexual purposes. This, and the reluctance to engage in routine breast care practices, could be considered factors, albeit ones that are difficult to quantify, in poor breast health.

Massage and hydrotherapy are gentle therapies, well suited for comfortable work on breast tissues, which enhance the efficiency of blood and lymph circulation. Scars and other types of fascial restrictions can be treated with techniques at which massage practitioners are highly skilled. Massage therapists are also expert at addressing the musculoskeletal causes which promote some of the pain and poor circulation in breasts. In many cases involving pain, congestion, edema, and restrictive or adhered scarring, massage therapy may be the treatment of choice.

As well, a trusted massage therapist can be of help to a woman who feels uneasy about having her breasts treated and palpated. The massage therapist can spend the time needed to talk with the client about her discomfort, and can approach the treatment gradually, ensuring that she is fully informed about what to expect. Her massage therapist is not someone a woman associates with fearful results and invasive or painful procedures, and consequently can be in a good position to help address the concerns which prevent many women from developing good breast health care habits.

So, while there are reasons why massage therapists hesitate to offer breast massage, there are also reasons why some therapists strongly advocate its use. Rather than avoiding breast massage training and practice, it may be that our wisest course is to work at eliminating any confusion that may exist between properly applied, indicated massage therapy and sexual misconduct. In openly promoting breast massage therapy, the responsibilities we assume are the proper training of massage practitioners and the articulation and enforcement of high standards of professional behaviour.

In the upcoming sections we will look at skills development and guidelines for massage therapists who are interested in learning about breast treatment and offering it to their clients.

Another concern about the tendency of massage therapists not to do breast massage is that this reluctance usually also leads to avoidance of a much larger area of tissue in the vicinity of the breasts. Several muscles and fascial structures which are frequently involved in stress-related syndromes, postural problems, and conditions of circulatory and neural compression are immediately adjacent to the breast. Massage therapists are often hesitant to properly access and treat these structures. It is quite common for the lateral and anterior chest to be avoided altogether.

Breast Massage Indications and Contraindications

Indications

congestion, edema, lymphedema

painful breasts

discomforts of pregnancy, breastfeeding, weaning

general drainage problems (family tendency, large breasts, etc.)

premenstrual congestion

tenderness and congestion related to benign conditions and changes associated with involution

following diagnostic procedures and recent surgeries, symptomatic relief and promotion of good quality scarring

breast trauma

restrictive, adhered, poorly oriented scars

reduction of pectoralis major tone following submuscular implant placement

discomforts related to cancer treatment*

integration of post-surgical changes, helping the client become comfortable with her body

education in self examination, self massage

client request for breast massage

client has a personal goal of becoming more comfortable with her breasts and having them touched

client wants assistance in breast monitoring

Contraindications

lactational mastitis, post-surgical infection, current active infection for any reason

specific on-site work at the location of an undiagnosed lump

specific on-site work at the location of an abscess

use of closed capsulotomy, or any other forceful technique attempting to reduce implant-related contracture

direct pressure on an implanted breast manifesting a distorted contour

implanted breast with submuscular placement manifesting lateral breast and subscapular pain (possible serratus anterior rupture)

client cannot, for whatever reason, clarify her wishes and comfortable boundaries

therapist cannot, for whatever reason, establish professional neutrality

client and therapist cannot, for whatever reason, establish open communication

client does not give consent, or withdraws consent

When treating a client with breast cancer, the therapist must have a body of knowledge about cancer, cancer therapies, and implications for massage treatment planning. Breast cancer does not have unique properties in these respects, so the subject is not covered in a breast-specific way in this book. The interested reader is referred to Curties, D., 'Massage Therapy and Cancer', Curties-Overzet Publications, 1998.

Summary of Specific Considerations in Breast Massage

1. Breast tissue is present beyond the visible contours of the breast. The tissue which extends beyond the rounded breast structure is equally likely to experience congestion and tenderness, or to develop benign or malignant formations.

2. There are no muscles or dense connective tissue structures in the breast; manual techniques employed by the practitioner should not overstress the breast's supporting fascial membranes and ligaments of Cooper.

3. It is not uncommon for a woman's two breasts to differ in size and shape; as well, some women have a visible amount of breast tissue in the axilla.

4. A percentage of breast pain results from causes outside the breast, usually musculoskeletal causes of ischemia or pain referral.

5. Males get breast conditions, too, including cancer. While the incidence is low, prognosis is often poor because of late diagnosis. Practitioner awareness is important.

6. Regardless of the specific reason for giving breast massage, the therapist should be mindful of the larger goal of enhancing the client's positive relationship to her breasts and commitment to breast health practices.

7. It is important to keep in mind that the chest can be an emotionally charged body area. This awareness includes staying fully present for the client during the treatment, and working carefully and respectfully within the client's wishes and comfort zone.

8. Women experiencing breast discomfort will often not volunteer information about their symptoms. Case history questions which elicit this information are useful, even if breast massage is not intended, to assist the massage

therapist to choose comfortable positioning and to avoid aspects of treatment which might add to the breast discomfort.

9. Breast massage usually feels more integrated and holistic when it is incorporated with anterior trunk and abdominal massage.

10. It is normal for lactating mothers to express milk from their breasts, often without any stimulation if their breasts are full, and frequently in response to breast massage or lying in positions which compress the breasts.

11. Women with duct ectasia are likely to be uncomfortable with cold applications and lying prone.

12. Post breast surgery or trauma, routine precautions to avoid promoting infection, handling drainage tubes inappropriately, or placing overly early stress on healing tissues apply as they would in similar cases involving other body parts.

13. Surgery, trauma, radiation therapy, and implant placement may all result in temporary or permanent sensory changes in the breast. These changes can include lost, reduced, or irritable sensory responses, including phenomena like parasthesia, dysesthesia, and allodynia. These sensory abnormalities can be extensive or patchy and vary from client to client.

14. Post mastectomy, the tissue area of the former breast should always be approached with the same special consideration accorded breasts. As well, it is important to be aware that the removed breast can have an energetic and/or sensory presence for the woman, including 'phantom limb' phenomena like pain and itching.

15. The practitioner needs to have an awareness of breast implant obsolescence. This includes monitoring for signs of distortion, calcification, and fill extrusion. Implant breakdown is especially likely as it ages beyond 7 years. Increased caution with manual techniques is indicated.

Protection of the Client and Practitioner

There are two fundamentals which are the basis of protection of the client and the massage therapist in breast massage. They are the same as the underpinnings of the therapeutic relationship in general. One is respect for the rights and autonomy of the client, and the other is proper training of the therapist. Good training is essential in that it establishes an understanding of the need for professional boundaries and behaviours which are premised on serving the best interests of the client.

Professionalism is very important. The breast massage client will be especially sensitive to overly casual or overly formal behaviour on the part of the practitioner. The language used by the massage therapist, the handling of draping and other privacy matters, the way in which the practitioner addresses the client's rights and concerns, and the professional appearance of the therapist and the clinical setting will all have an impact on the client's feeling of safety.

Choice, for both the client and the practitioner, are also key to safety in breast massage. Given the sexual symbolism of breasts and the prevalence of abusive touch, it is understood, and must be respected, that some clients and some practitioners will never be comfortable with breast massage. Therapists who find themselves in this position must learn how to communicate their stance appropriately to their clients, and be able to make good referrals.

Massage therapy practitioners who are providing breast massage **must** be adequately trained. It is important to recognize that academic and hands-on learning are only one component of the training needed, and in this circumstance, not the most important component. Clients will bring a realm of different histories and comfort levels to the treatment situation, and these will be largely unrelated to the indicators for breast massage in the case. It is imperative that the practitioner has a good command of the skills of the therapeutic relationship, including clarifying and respecting the client's needs and objectives, communicating treatment information properly, obtaining consent, safeguarding the client's rights to safety and privacy, professional boundary setting, therapist self-monitoring, and appropriate referral.

In the realm of ethics and personal behaviour, what one sees and experiences is a more powerful influence than what one is told to believe or do. Incorporating breast massage into massage therapy training programs provides the opportunity to **show** students how professionals handle clinical situations which have special aspects. While it is true that education will not stop an individual with truly evil intent, experts in this kind of criminal behaviour largely acknowledge that stopping such a person is the role of the legal system. Fortunately, this type of individual is very much in the minority in our profession. Most of the cases of sexual misconduct which come to discipline proceedings in the massage therapy context reflect uninformed, misguided, or poorly boundaried behaviour on the part of the therapist.

Students need to give **and** receive breast massage. This obligation is part of the set of responsibilities of the bodywork student. Even though it will be a more onerous requirement for some, it is important to find ways to ensure that the learner experiences the treatment from the perspectives of both the client and the therapist. Despite the obvious differences, this is also true for male students. The trainer can help students who are uncomfortable by making sure they feel heard and have time to think and talk about their difficulties, allowing them to select their practice partners, giving dispensation to complete the requirement in a more private space and/or with additional time, and being open to setting up contracts for alternate arrangements. For example, the student could contract to observe only in class and to do the practical component as a project over which he or she can exercise more control. Under flexible conditions most students overcome their discomfort. The others gain a deeper understanding of what prevents them from achieving the ease they need to become capable practitioners in this area.

It is true that breast massage and other more highly charged types of treatment are handled better by some practitioners than others. If an instructor feels strongly that a student is not ready to assume the responsibilities involved, it is important to communicate this message clearly, explaining the reasons and advising additional training and/or self disqualification from giving the treatment in question.

Some advocate that breast massage should only be taught as advanced or postgraduate education. The merit in this position is that the learners self select and commit to the training specifically - they are not obliged to participate. As well, students at this level will have had basic training, hopefully other types of advanced education, and work experience, all of which help optimize their suitability. On the other hand, exposure to various types of treatment in massage school helps future therapists identify what interests them. It is also true that self selection is not always reliable. The school environment can provide consistency of instruction and learner monitoring over time, and gives the student a supportive setting in which to practice and seek out supervision as the need develops. The school also has more time and resources to oversee the additional practice or remedial work needed by some students.

The appropriateness of breast massage in undergraduate education may depend on the length and content of the school's program. Therapeutic relationship skills must be in place before breast massage is taught. There are many methods of achieving these skills, both within an undergraduate curriculum and outside of it, but a well designed training program of good duration creates an environment of consistent reinforcement. Trainers in breast massage have a responsibility to see that their students have the necessary prior learning.

Massage therapists and educators must also be aware of the legislative and regulatory environments in their jurisdictions. Breast massage is generally accepted practice in Canada, with some provinces specifying guidelines related to its use. In the United States, the situation varies greatly state by state - some states have clear guidelines about breast massage, some do not regulate it at all, and in some states breast massage is actually illegal.

The therapist's good sense, or common sense, is important to the success and safety of breast massage. Although paranoia is not completely unjustified, we should not be ruled by it. The reality is that when the massage therapist is comfortable and trustworthy, the client is likely to be fine. In the subsections which follow, we will address the elements which influence the actions and decision-making of the therapist, and form the basis of a therapeutic relationship in which both the practitioner and the client are well protected.

Therapist Self Awareness and Self Monitoring

While empathy, good intentions, and a sincere desire to help people are important requisites for the massage therapist, they are not enough to ensure client protection. Our ability to participate in a therapeutic relationship which provides safety to both parties hinges on our capacity to make a clear separation between our own needs and interests and those of our clients.

Therapists and clients can have the same goals and similar points of view about many things, but we are fundamentally different entities in the therapeutic relationship. The person who is being touched on multiple levels through treatment, while unclothed and lying down in a private room with one other clothed, upright person present, is by definition at a power disadvantage. Whether or not the massage therapist feels more powerful in the situation, the power differential exists.

When breast treatment is added to this equation, more dynamics come into play. For example, a client may directly or indirectly seek approval of her breasts, stemming from a deep-seated sense of their inadequacy. Is a massage therapist in a position to give such approval? What would that mean to their therapeutic relationship?

If the 'wounded healer' theories have validity, many of us bring to our career choice a need to heal elements in our own histories involving personal boundaries. These needs can manifest in caretakers in specific ways. Perhaps three of the most likely are: excessive investment in how the client feels and is progressing, 'overgiving' of oneself through not setting healthy limits, and wanting to 'make' the client better so that we can feel needed and validated. There is a fine line, vitally important to find, between being a caring and effective practitioner with an intact ego and someone who gets personal validation needs met inappropriately through the client-therapist relationship.

Each of us is on our own path, uniquely ours, and needs to have this fact understood and supported as we make choices and live our lives as best we can. One of the most significant things a health care practitioner can do for a client is to keep sight of this pivotal truth. The therapist's personal motivations and sense of work satisfaction, while certainly related to success in helping people feel better, must come from other factors as well. When a practitioner can clearly understand what he or she 'gets' from being a massage therapist in the way of personal growth and development, an enjoyable independent workstyle, learning about the fascinations of how the human body works, meeting interesting people from all walks of life, and so on, the motivation to be a good helper stays in perspective.

As we all know, none of us is perfect - maintaining balance as a caregiver is an ongoing challenge. We make mistakes with certain situations and certain clients. The practitioner's central skill is in thinking and re-thinking situations, recognizing personal weak spots, acknowledging and correcting errors, and striving to grow in maturity and humility. The client's best interests are paramount. As we work with people we have to discipline ourselves to stay focused on this fact. This does not mean that we should be self-sacrificing in a martyred way, but rather that when a choice has to be made between following our own agendas and inclinations and being responsible for doing the right thing, it is our job and our sacred trust to do the right thing.

In the breast massage context, it is easy to stumble. Here are a few examples of well-meaning practitioners who may be losing perspective on what the client herself needs:

Therapist 1

Natalie is very comfortable with her body and her breasts. She is a fit former dancer who went into massage therapy as a natural extension of being an athlete. Her client Clarissa is a 58 year old woman who has been struggling for several years with breast cancer and has had a number of problems with the implant placed after her mastectomy. Clarissa is depressed and discouraged as she contemplates another surgery to remove the implant. Natalie feels that it would be healthy for Clarissa to feel more angry about what has been done to her body.

Therapist 2

John is a caring and sensitive male whose new client Maria has a painful sexual abuse history. They get along well, and over time she confides some of the details of her personal story. John starts to consider the possibility that by giving Maria breast massage he can help her see that there are men who are capable of touching her without being abusive.

Therapist 3

Lucy is a very maternal kind of person with 4 children of her own who enjoys taking care of her clients. About half of her massage therapy practice consists of women who are pregnant or have just had babies. Rebecca begins coming to see Lucy when she is 8 months pregnant. Rebecca is a young unmarried model with a beautiful face and body who did not intend to get pregnant and didn't realize she was until a late-stage abortion would have been necessary. Although Rebecca has now adjusted to the pregnancy, she is adamant that she does not intend to breastfeed. Her principal interest in receiving breast massage is to help avoid stretch marks. Lucy sets out to convince Rebecca that breastfeeding is more important than how her breasts look.

These scenarios are rich with the human elements common to massage practice. We can see both positive and potentially harmful aspects in the stances the practitioners seem poised to take. We hope that each of them thinks carefully before proceeding: Is this my need or hers? Am I imposing my own history or values on this client? Could I be adding to her burden by following my inclination? Why do I feel as strongly as I do? Have I uncovered a trigger of my own here? Am I overly invested in taking care of this client? Do I have a need to get her to see things my way? What course would I take if I were trying to think only of what is best for her?

None of us is sure what is best for the clients in the above scenarios. In each instance the therapist's instincts could be exactly right or painfully wrong, damaging the therapeutic relationship and perhaps causing harm to the client. The therapist who has good self awareness and self monitoring skills has a very good chance of working out the best path; the practitioner without these skills travels a much more bumpy road and may actually be quite destructive.

Our personal blind spots are very difficult to take into account, and are therefore most likely to cause problems as we seek to care for others. We all require help becoming responsible and trustworthy practitioners. Massage therapists need to embrace the challenges of continuous self development as part of our commitment to our work. Assuming that confidentiality is being properly maintained, it is healthy to talk about personally difficult work situations. Peer supervision groups can provide an excellent venue for reflecting on our cases with colleagues. Personal psychotherapy and professional supervision relationships can also be very important resources.

As practitioners, it is essential that we be watchful for indicators which can alert us to the need for some self reflection. We each have our problem areas, and must try to recognize them in clinical practice scenarios that arise. While our inclinations may be 'right' or 'wrong' or even immaterial in the end, the discipline of self reflection will help determine the best course or the best method for proceeding.

Indicators common to most of us include:

1. feeling very strongly about the direction a client should take or the outcome that should occur

2. feeling angry or frustrated with a client, needing to make a case that the client is at fault

3. not wanting to see a client any more; not staying 'present' during a client's treatments

4. feeling unable or unwilling to talk a situation over with a client

5. seeing oneself or a friend or family member in the client

6. feeling that the situation is familiar, something one knows all about

7. wanting to mother or 'heal' the client

8. not wanting to talk a dilemma over with anyone, deciding to keep it private

9. making too many accommodations

10. enjoying being put on a pedestal by a client

11. finding a client very appealing or attractive, acting 'lovestruck'

12. acquiescing on important matters rather than doing what is right or therapeutically best

13. revealing too much non-relevant personal information

14. finding oneself acting like an authority in the situation, doing 'I am the professional'

15. strongly needing something from a client or fostering a client's sense of needing you

The practitioner may find that there are certain cases and situations that he or she just cannot handle professionally. In the list of therapist comments at the beginning of this chapter, one woman states that because of the deaths of several people close to her from breast cancer she cannot achieve professional neutrality about breast massage. The fact that she sees the problem is key. She may choose to work on this issue personally until she reaches a point where she can be comfortable offering breast treatment, or she may decide never to do breast massage, but her awareness will help her to avoid harming her clients. A massage therapist with a personal history of sexual abuse may encounter a similar set of difficulties.

The practitioner must also be able to desexualize the client-therapist relationship and the breast massage situation. There are no shades of grey here. While human beings find each other attractive and sexual arousal is certainly a natural occurrence, it is **not** something over which we have no control. Sexual energy entering a therapeutic relationship is always cause for concern and reflection. This is a power imbalance relationship in which acting on sexual inclinations can cause both parties tremendous harm. A therapist should be concerned about fantasizing about a client, finding massaging a particular client arousing, or getting 'in love' kinds of feelings. Practitioners can be especially susceptible to getting into this type of trouble when their personal lives are not going well. While consciously knowing better, they may subconsciously start using their clients as sources of comfort, approval, and reinforcement. Such a therapist needs to recognize that he or she has gone off course and establish a path of self correction, seeking support and guidance as needed.

The 'centred' practitioner will also be able to respond with appropriate boundaries in place if a client expresses an attraction or talks about finding breast massage arousing. The massage therapist needs to communicate in an unconfused, compassionate way that the purpose of the treatment is not intended to be seductive or sexual, and that it is not comfortable to continue if the client is in any way mistaken about this. The therapist needs to be clear internally in order to give this message in a simple, honest manner.

Working with more private or vulnerable body areas requires that the therapist be especially alert and responsive. Being 'present' helps protect against the inadvertent creation of an environment which the client could experience as unsafe. The practitioner needs to self monitor for levels of upset or distractedness which might cause problems. It is better to communicate about feeling unwell or not being focused enough to give breast treatment on a particular day than to set up an atmosphere which the client may feel uneasy about or misinterpret.

Excessive sensitivity or solicitude can also be problematic. It can be misread in various ways, and it can also be annoying. A calm, matter-of-fact, empathetic approach which stays in fairly good tune with the type of atmosphere the client prefers for the treatment is what works best.

Given the possibility that breast massage clients may experience strong psychoemotional reactions, the massage therapist needs to feel comfortable and adequate handling emotional release. It is not acceptable to panic or emotionally abandon the client. Training is important here - there are various courses and programs which can assist therapists to enhance their skill and comfort levels. This is an area where practitioners can sometimes feel particularly disconcerted or triggered, necessitating personal work on their part. In general terms, it is wise to pursue at least a basic level of skill in handling somatoemotional release, because even though it is possible not to offer breast massage, emotional release reactions are not limited to breast treatment.

Male Practitioners

It would be wrong to suggest that a properly trained male massage therapist cannot give appropriate breast treatment to a consenting client. Disqualification purely on the grounds of gender, although advocated by many for obvious reasons, cannot really be defended. If a male therapist is the practitioner a client chooses and trusts, it makes sense for him to provide indicated breast treatment, assuming he is comfortable doing so. Factors like his being the only qualified practitioner available can also arise, especially in non-urban areas.

It is true, however, that the male practitioner may be more closely scrutinized for behaviour and intention, and could be more at risk over mistakes made.

The topics discussed in this section on protection of the client and practitioner could be said to apply in greater measure to the male massage therapist. He must be especially careful in his client-therapist interactions and boundary-setting, and very clear in his personal self monitoring and communication of intent. He also needs to be alert for signs that a client's interest in him or in breast treatment may be more complex than meets the eye.

It is possible that a client may be more susceptible to re-traumatization through receiving breast massage from a male therapist. The concern that a client may be re-traumatized by bodywork should be a factor in decision-making for all massage therapists, and the risk can at times be very difficult to assess. In the case of breast massage, the male practitioner will need to become as knowledgeable as he can about the client's history and goals and carefully consider the impact receiving breast massage from him might have. An honest, straightforward expression of this concern may help engage the client in a good conversation about the risks for her. If the client is working with a psychotherapist, it is an excellent idea to request that they carefully consider the pros and cons together.

It is perhaps best if the male practitioner assumes that he will not be a client's first choice for breast massage. He should have a referral list on hand so that he can offer alternatives to clients who need breast work. One must become reconciled to the fact that sometimes someone else is the best therapist for the job. This maturity and sense of responsibility is particularly required of male practitioners when breast massage is being considered.

If the client chooses to proceed with him, the therapist may decide to take additional precautions, such as using written consent forms and recording having given her breast massage informational materials.

The male therapist's personal and professional maturity will be scrutinized during his interactions with clients considering breast massage. His trustworthiness must be evident and well communicated. He needs to avoid behaviours which could be interpreted as pressuring or judgemental or signals of sexual interest. Nevertheless, if he feels comfortable with breast massage and with the client, if he makes clear his willingness to refer to a female practitioner, if he accepts the client's decisions and can work within her comfort indicators, and if he has her informed consent, the male massage therapist can proceed as any practitioner would.

When the Client has a Sexual Abuse History

Most massage therapists are not expert in working with sexual abuse, and yet we encounter it regularly in the course of our work. Many practitioners also have personal sexual abuse histories and are in various stages of coming to terms with and healing the past. While it is not within the massage therapy scope of practice to be primary care practitioners in this area, we need to be aware and comfortable enough to be able to create safety for our clients in the massage therapy setting.

Treating clients with sexual abuse histories is of particular concern in the context of offering breast massage. There are two primary fears: the risk of re-traumatizing the client, and the possibility of increased peril of becoming entangled in misconduct or sexual abuse allegations. These are both important concerns.

There are counterbalancing considerations, however. Massage therapists work daily with individuals who have been sexually traumatized, sometimes knowing they are doing so and sometimes not. It is not a circumstance that can always be 'chosen'. The strongest safeguard is never to massage known victims of sexual abuse or treat high risk body parts like breasts. This is not foolproof, but it does increase the practitioner's margin of safety. As a guiding principle, however, it is not very consistent with the values and responsibilities of our profession.

It is also true that some clients come to massage therapists specifically for help in 'normalizing' their experience of being touched. It is often vitally important to their happiness and personal wellbeing. The therapist who is well prepared for such a challenge is sometimes able to do tremendous service.

Working with sexual abuse requires psychotherapeutic intervention. Touch is an extremely powerful tool in this arena. Knowing the limits of one's expertise helps prevent getting in over one's head and placing oneself and the client at risk of harm. It is generally best for clients grappling with sexual abuse issues to be working with a team of health professionals. Massage therapy, which adds the intense stimulus of touch, is not usually the first therapeutic direction chosen. In fact, introducing massage would ideally always be done with a great deal of prior thought and with psychotherapeutic supervision. The psychotherapist can provide support and 'debriefing', suggesting appropriate treatment guidelines, sorting out reactions from receiving massage, and helping safeguard the client's sense of autonomy and safety. The psychotherapist can also be a resource for the massage practitioner to assist in decision-making about the massage therapy plan. While this ideal circumstance is not always feasible, providing massage therapy within the parameters of the client's psychotherapy treatment plan can offer a great deal of protection to both the client and the massage therapist.

The advisability of treating potentially highly triggering body parts like breasts must be considered very carefully in light of the client's status, objectives, and support system. Timing can also be critical - introducing breast massage, no matter how indicated, is a very sensitive decision.

A client's awareness of past sexual abuse and understanding of its implications are not always in place prior to starting massage therapy. Massage practitioners can be understandably reluctant to insist that a client takes a major step like beginning psychotherapy. Clearly, the handling of any discussions on this subject requires diplomacy and skill. However, clients generally do appreciate it, at the time or subsequently, when a practitioner acts to safeguard their best interests. The massage therapist is wise not to proceed with some or all forms of treatment, especially modalities like breast massage, if it seems that the client may need a support system which is not in place. This dialogue or negotiation will sometimes ensue over a period of time after massage therapy has begun; in this case the client may experience first-hand the need for additional therapies. Ultimately, it is the responsibility of the practitioner to guarantee basic protections in the therapeutic relationship. When a client shows signs which may signify unrecognized or unacknowledged sexual abuse issues, and a treatment like breast massage is being considered, there can be significant risk of harm from getting into a situation which neither the practitioner nor the client may be well equipped to handle.

With someone who has experienced sexual abuse and is engaged in a healing process, the role of the massage therapist is to support the therapeutic journey through helping the client to experience safe touch in a relationship of boundaried caring. Each client's personal story is unique and will involve individual memories, traumas, and sensitivities. Even so, there are some considerations which repeatedly arise in working with clients who have sexual abuse histories. An awareness of needs and behaviour patterns that can be common to such clients can help the practitioner avoid making naive errors, especially in decisions about whether or not to proceed with breast treatment.

1. The client may have difficulty defining and enforcing personal boundaries. This frequently manifests in feeling unable or unentitled to say no to being touched. This difficulty can compromise the consent dialogue, and may be an ongoing feature in the therapeutic relationship.

   The practitioner can help by being very alert for non-verbal indicators of discomfort, and by doing everything possible to encourage the client's expression of treatment preferences. The massage therapist is often wise to diplomatically but directly address the concern that the client may be reluctant to express choices and wishes, and could therefore leave them both open to the making of painful mistakes. When the client communicates comfort requirements, no matter how indirectly, the massage therapist must strive to notice and acknowledge them and make every effort to work within them. These can include preferences about positioning, extent of undressing, a need to keep talking during the treatment, and so on.

I am reminded of a poignant incident relayed by the instructor of a course I took on therapeutic relationship skills. A massage therapist, talking to a new client before her first treatment, gestured to the carefully made up massage table and told her to undress and get on the table, asking that she call out when she was ready. There was no call for several minutes, so the therapist knocked and heard a faint "Come in." On entering the room, she was stunned to see the client lying naked on top of the table with her fists clenched and eyes tightly closed. The therapist said gently "I'm really sorry. I made a mistake. I forgot you haven't had massage before. I meant to tell you to remove any clothes you feel comfortable taking off and then lie under the top sheet and blanket. I'll leave again and let you get ready." When she re-entered the room, the therapist found that the client had replaced all her clothing except her socks and had pulled the cover sheet up over her chin.

2. The client may have a strong need to control what happens during the treatment. Some clients manifest the opposite tendency to that described in #1 above, wanting to tightly control every aspect of what the practitioner does. Since the massage therapist will tend

to find this conduct annoying, it helps to have an understanding of what may lie behind it. This type of behaviour may also act as an early signal that a new client has experienced personal boundary violations of some type.

It is important to be aware that clients with sexual trauma histories can be expressing healthy and healing tendencies through taking this type of control. In most safe and trusting therapeutic relationships the client and practitioner can negotiate ways of communicating and proceeding that satisfy the client and are workable for the therapist.

3. The client may behave in an overtly sexual manner, for example flirting and being charming, moving in ways that expose body parts, sexualizing the massage, revealing intimate personal anecdotes, placing excessive value on body attractiveness, and so on. This can make for some disconcerting moments for the massage therapist. These behaviours, inappropriate in the massage setting, generally stem from self esteem damage which leads the person to believe that sexual currency is the only tool that is going to work or be of value in getting approval and attention. It is crucial that the massage therapist maintains very clear boundaries, but in a way that offers alternative types of respect and caring.

Responding in kind to the behaviour is risky for the therapist and potentially damaging to the therapeutic relationship. It is not professionally sound behaviour and may reproduce elements of the client's previous traumatizing situation.

4. The client may experience memories, flashbacks, and emotional reactions of various kinds. The client may also regress, speaking and acting in ways that are more in keeping with previous experiences than the current reality of the treatment. The massage therapist may take on a role or persona in the client's view which reflects parts of such experiences. These responses can be challenging to work with and may create some jeopardy for the practitioner. The client's emotional reactions can range from deep distress to anger to shock to depression.

There are no simple guidelines for the practitioner who finds himself or herself in such circumstances with a client. Many need to make use of their personal and professional support systems, and perhaps to seek out additional training. The client's psychotherapy relationship can also function as a strong anchor at these times. Although it is true that practitioner errors can be costly, it is also true that in a well contained situation with proper supports, clients and massage therapists can find ways to work well together through these experiences. The best situation, of course, is to be well trained and well matured as a therapist before consciously choosing to work with this type of client. When circumstances occur outside this ideal, the practitioner who has a strong grasp of the guiding principles of the client-therapist relationship, and the capacity to communicate and self monitor with honesty and integrity, will be able to take steps to protect both self and client while they decide together how best to cope with the unplanned or unexpected.

Breast Massage as a Standard Treatment Practice?

Massage therapists must communicate the message that all body parts are equally valued and accepted, even though there is selectivity about how or if they are touched. Automatic inclusion of breasts in full body treatment, while it may make sense in the abstract from a holistic perspective, is not workable in our societal context.

For general relaxation massage at this point in time, massaging the breasts is not necessary, and probably not even conducive, to the achievement of treatment goals. We have no physiological data about the non-specific (generalized) effects of breast massage. Given the powerful sociosexual overlay in North America[104], common sense dictates that for most clients who have not specifically requested breast work, relaxation is unlikely to be one. In many jurisdictions (Ontario is an example), breast massage is excluded from general treatment protocols and considered a type of treatment which must be specifically requested and for which specific consent must be given.

It is worth noting that cultural differences exist in attitudes toward breast massage. Many European clients, for example, both male and female, are astounded at our cautious avoidance of the chest area.

In the ordinary course of events, breast massage is given because it has been recommended by the massage therapist or perhaps another health care practitioner. Some clients, however, identify a need for breast massage and request it as part of their massage therapy treatment plan. Some prefer the completeness of a full body treatment which includes breast massage. In these circumstances, assuming the practitioner is in agreement, there can be no objection.

Communication and Trust

Nothing ensures the protection of the client and practitioner like the establishment of a therapeutic relationship in which there is trust and good communication. Trust does not come automatically - it needs to be built and earned. It is our responsibility to demonstrate our trustworthiness and our willingness to engage with our clients in dialogue about their needs, concerns, and goals. Once this trust has been established, the client is more likely to be relaxed and flexible about new concepts like breast treatment.

Communication is not just about information. During these introductory conversations, the therapist's demonstration of reliability in being caring, 'present', and responsive to her concerns helps persuade the client that the ongoing character of the relationship will be one in which she can place her trust. Non-verbal communication is also very powerful, especially in the context of a sensitive matter like breast massage. The client senses for elements in the therapist's professional presentation which inspire confidence. Honesty, integrity, and accountability are communicated on subtle as well as overt levels.

Massage therapy is a relative newcomer in the public mindset, and most people have questions about what to expect. This is especially true about breast massage. We need to provide women with information about what breast massage can offer them without pushing, judging, or rushing their decision.

Most women want to know how their personal choices and need for privacy will be incorporated into the breast treatment plan. Such conversations should outline information about positioning, draping, and techniques and modalities commonly used. It is important to identify options the client has with respect to these treatment components. Specific boundaries, such as the fact that the nipple and areola will not be touched, should also be included.

These discussions do not need to be extended, and do not have to be completed all at once, but they should include the following key elements: why the treatment is indicated, what to expect, the client's rights and choices, and the practitioner's willingness to abide by her wishes and only proceed when and if she is ready.

Communication is key to ensuring that the preferences of the client and the intentions of the therapist are understood. Both the practitioner and the client must make the effort to clarify their comfort and safety needs. **A client who cannot, for whatever reason, participate in such a conversation in order to inform herself and communicate her boundaries should not receive breast massage.** There simply isn't adequate protection for her or for her therapist in this situation.

Similarly, **the practitioner who cannot talk openly and fully about the proposed treatment must consider himself or herself unsuited to work with a client who needs breast massage.** The client cannot be properly informed in this situation. Also, proceeding with a therapist who is this uncomfortable is not safe. Indirectly communicated discomfort manifests in various ways. The therapist's feelings and intentions become open to misinterpretation. This can be especially true if a client brings to the situation a history or predisposition which can result in her personal issues becoming superimposed on unclear messages from the therapist.

If a client decides against having breast massage, her decision must be received with equanimity. Once the topic has been discussed and a 'no' conclusion reached, the therapist can indicate openness to having the subject raised again in future if the client wishes, and then must move on.

It is important to consider the best use of language when talking about breasts and breast work. While there are many slang terms for breasts in common usage, they are not usually appropriate in a professional setting. It is not a matter of being prudish - the clinical atmosphere often becomes less formal as a client and therapist get to know each other over time. However, the use of terms which may strike a client as inappropriate can give her the wrong impression of the seriousness with which the therapist views the boundaries she needs in place to feel comfortable. It is best to err on the side of caution in these respects.

Sometimes clients express concerns about the size or attractiveness of their breasts. It is natural to want to be helpful and encouraging, and to support all women to feel confident in their unique sensuality. At the same time, as therapists we have to be cautious about expressing what could be taken as a personal opinion about a client's breasts. Safety for both participants in the therapeutic relationship is jeopardized if the situation begins to take on sexual elements.

From the other point of view, we do not want to create a negative inference in the way we respond or do not respond to remarks clients make about their breasts. We don't want to shut down a client's wish to explore body image issues. These conversations involve situation-specific judgements. Sometimes it is best to respond in a warm, general way initially and to return to the topic later when the therapeutic relationship has been established for a while and there is trust and comfortable familiarity.

One of the advantages of good training is that it assists the therapist in understanding the dynamics of the therapeutic relationship. It provides a safe zone in which the learner can make mistakes and can struggle with personal dilemmas impeding his or her ability to respond to clients with clear and open communication. It is best to begin this type of preparation in advance in order to avoid 'practising' communication basics on clients in highly charged situations like breast massage. In the absence of good school-based training, or along with it, establishing a supervision or psychotherapeutic relationship can assist the practitioner to achieve better self awareness and to build therapeutic relationship skills.

Most Women Need Time to Think about Breast Massage

In instances where breast massage has caused problems, the client will often report having had the treatment 'sprung on her'. She gave consent in the moment, but on reflection felt that she had been caught off guard and was not happy with either herself or the practitioner. While consent was strictly speaking obtained, the therapeutic relationship may have been irretrievably damaged.

It is important to recognize that women need time to consider whether they are open to receiving breast massage. Some will have done this thinking in advance, but most will encounter breast treatment as a concept for the first time when it is suggested by their massage therapist. Given our particular societal relationship to breasts, the therapist should not assume that a client will be ready to receive breast massage on the day it is first discussed. In fact, it is probably safest to develop a reticence about moving forward on the same day, even if the client appears to readily agree.

Conversation is also not necessarily the best avenue for introducing the idea. Some clients just do not want to have this conversation, and are not open to receiving breast massage. There are many simple ways to put the possibility forward and give clients the option of expressing interest or definite disinterest. For example:

- incorporate breast health and breast massage questions in your case history form (see samples in the box which follows)
- have a brochure about breast massage in your waiting area
- display your certificate of completion of a breast massage advanced training course
- create a new client orientation kit with an inclusion (brochure or article) about breast massage and/or an invitation to ask questions on the subject if interested

Sample Questions to Incorporate in a General Case History Form or Client Intake Questionnaire

___ Breast Pain

___ Diagnosed Breast Condition
Pls. Specify_____

___ Breast Implants
Type:_____
How Long Ago?_____
Any Problems?_____
Pls. Specify_____

___ Breast Surgery
Type:_____
How Long Ago?_____
Any problems?_____
Pls. Specify_____

Are you familiar with breast massage? _____

Are you interested in discussing breast massage or receiving reading material about it? _____
    If yes, pls. specify:_____

If you have a condition that might benefit from breast massage, would you like more information about this treatment? Do you have any questions or concerns about breast massage that you would like to mention here?
(I will follow up with you.)

_____
_____

Are there any parts of your body you do not want massaged?

_____

If comfortable, pls. give a brief reason here:

_____

Would you be comfortable if I raised this issue in conversation with you?

_____

Genitals are never massaged, but breasts are sometimes treated if indicated and the woman gives specific consent. Do you have any interest in talking about breast treatment at this time?

_____

The interested and completely disinterested client alike often prefer being given an opening to express themselves in their own way. A case history form answer can be helpful in giving the therapist a clear signal from many female clients, and may be the only communication that is needed. Often clients will absorb the fact that you offer breast massage and raise the subject at some time in the future if they develop a need or become more comfortable with the idea.

Most practitioners, whether intentionally or not, are secretive about offering breast massage. As a result, they only approach clients in direct conversation to suggest breast treatment, and rely on their 'gut instinct' about who might be amenable to having this treatment offered. Some therapists put forward a strong 'should' message, generating an excessive intensity in the conversation which in part reflects the practitioner's need to ensure that the client understands that breast massage really is indicated in her case. These conversations will go awry with some clients despite the massage therapist's best instincts and intentions. It is also very significant that therapists avoid approaching numbers of women who could perhaps benefit tremendously from breast massage out of uncertainty about how they will react. Inclusion of the subject of breast massage in the ordinary methods used to inform clients, or to seek information from them, allows for a more neutral introduction of the idea to one's larger client base, and provides a measure of certainty for the practitioner beyond gut feelings.

In preliminary conversations with clients, it is important not to push breast massage, or to become defensive about why it is offered. Initial emotional reactions usually concentrate on concerns about safety and choice. Try to hear and respond to the concern being expressed and the need of the client at that moment.

> *"I saw your Breast Massage certificate on the wall. I want you to know I don't want anything like that."*

> *"That's fine, Moira. I would never do anything without your consent."*
>   .....

"My sister has been getting breast massage from you for a while now. I have to admit I don't understand why anyone would want breast massage."

"Breasts have health needs and problems like other tissues, and massage therapy can be very effective when a woman has breast pain, congestion, or swelling. There are other more serious circumstances, too, where breast massage can be helpful, like surgery or cancer. Some women like the holistic feel of having their breasts included in a full body massage.

Would you like some information to take home? I'm happy to talk with you about breast massage, either now, or after you've had a chance to read some things that I can give you on the subject. But receiving breast massage is a personal choice. It really is up to you."

.....

"I've just been reading the breast massage brochure in your waiting room. I've had pain in my left breast since I had a biopsy 4 years ago. I've never thought about getting breast massage for it - I'm not sure I'm entirely comfortable with the idea, but I haven't found anything else that works. Can you tell me what breast massage would be like and if you think it would work for me?"

"Massage may be able to help reduce the pain in your breast by making the scar more pliable and less stuck to the tissues around it. I could give you a better opinion after taking a look at it. When you say you aren't entirely comfortable with the idea of breast massage, you aren't alone. Why don't you take home this literature and think about it? I also have some clients who have told me they are happy to discuss their breast massage experiences with women who have questions. If you'd like a couple of names and phone numbers, I can easily provide them. Give me a call, or we'll talk some more next session - once you've had time to consider. I'd be happy to treat your breast, but only when you feel certain you are comfortable to go ahead with it."

In situations where you believe the client's symptoms warrant advocating breast massage in her case, the same basic guidelines apply.

> *"Jacqui, Now that you are pregnant and your breasts are really tender, I thought about raising the idea of breast massage with you. On the case history form you filled out when you first started coming here you stated that you weren't interested in having your breasts treated. If you still feel that way, that's perfectly fine. But if you'd like, I can talk about what massage therapy can offer you while you are pregnant and breastfeeding. I'm not suggesting working on your breasts today, but if you want to discuss breast massage, or would like some information to read at home... etc."*

If you are the one initiating the subject of breast massage, make sure the client understands your reasons for raising the subject. This is a simple matter of briefly describing the indications in her case. Do not have a "Have you ever thought about having your breasts massaged? No? Okay." conversation. The problem with this unclear exchange is that the woman (along with others to whom she may relay the exchange) is left to contemplate what lay behind your question.

As you can see, the massage therapist needs to have several items on hand: a good general case history form, a new client orientation kit, an informational brochure* about breast massage, a portfolio of references/articles/excerpts from books such as this, and so on! At minimum, a few of these items are essential. A list of names of clients open to discussing their experiences with breast massage is also very helpful. Sometimes you will find doctors or other health practitioners in your community who are willing to vouch for you and the viability of breast massage. Having these resources pre-organized and readily available assists you in introducing the idea of breast treatment, in informing clients about breast massage in a way that reinforces its legitimacy, and in providing women with the time and 'space' to talk to others and privately consider their options.

* *Create your own brochure, or enquire with the publisher of this book about ordering ours.*

Consent

Massage therapists are responsible for ensuring that our clients are fully exercising their right to informed consent. The components of informed consent are as follows:

- The client understands the nature of the proposed treatment and the reasons for it.

- The client understands the components of the proposed treatment plan, namely body parts to be included, proposed draping and positioning, modalities to be used, how much pain might be experienced, the expected duration of the treatment plan, and so on.

- The client's stated goals and wishes are in alignment with the proposed treatment.

- The client is aware of the types of treatment reactions that might be experienced.

- The client understands that he or she can stop the treatment or request changes in the treatment plan at any time.

- The client states a clear 'yes' to the plan.

These elements of consent apply across the board in massage therapy treatment. They are not different for breast massage, but their application is perhaps a bit more stringent. For example, when a client gives consent for a standard full body relaxation massage, or treatment of a sprained ankle, the expectations of the therapist and the client are reasonably well aligned at the outset. The specifics covered in the consent discussion, though fundamentally important, are usually fairly routine. Breast massage, like treatment of other body parts understood to involve more emotional vulnerability and privacy considerations, cannot begin with the assumption that the client and therapist both know what to expect.

In addition to the components of good pre-consent communication discussed in previous sections, it is very important to acknowledge the psychoemotional aspects of breast massage. Breast treatment may cause a client to have strong emotional responses or a return of uncomfortable memories. All potential breast massage clients need to know that, while you are not predicting or expecting any particular reaction, such responses to breast work can happen. If a woman is aware that she has emotionally painful associations with her breasts, it must be her choice to go forward knowing that these issues may come to the surface during or after her treatments. Many clients have the inclination and personal resources to work with their traumatic experiences in ways that are healing and meaningful for them, but if they haven't thought about the possibility that breast massage could propel them into such personal places, they are less likely to feel ready to handle them well. In other words, they may believe that they are giving consent to something expected to take place on a more superficial level than ultimately occurs.

It is also important to acknowledge that people with sexual abuse histories may be inclined to give consent too readily. If you have specific information about a client's background, these comments can be carefully adapted to her situation. If not, they can be mentioned in a more universal context. The number of women who have had coercive sexual experiences is quite large, and those who do not have such a background are still likely to acknowledge the importance of really feeling ready before giving consent to breast treatment.

Breast massage cannot be included in any type of blanket consent protocol. It must be consented to separately and specifically. The client should have absolute clarity about her right to suggest modifications, to choose not to receive the treatment on any given day, or to discontinue breast massage at any time. Consent for breast massage must be renewed before each session.

Therapists sometimes feel that discussions about consent can be time-consuming, awkward, or overly formal. This is really more an issue of practising until the therapist has evolved the dialogue to a point of personal ease. As long as the elements of informed consent are included and consent is obtained before treatment begins, the client and practitioner can handle their discussions in any time frame or manner that works for them.

Some therapists prefer to seek written consent for breast massage. This is certainly a viable option, but it is important not to present it in a 'heavy' or ominous way. The consent form should include the elements listed above, and be signed and dated. If written consent is being used, it must be adapted if the treatment plan changes. Therapists who do not require signed consent should always protect themselves by entering the date and nature of the breast massage verbal consent agreement into their client record.

Finding a Lump

The moment when a massage therapist finds a new or potentially ominous tissue formation in a client's breast is another time when the practitioner's handling of the situation has the potential to damage the client's trust and wellbeing. The magnitude of breast cancer fear felt by most women makes it difficult for clients to have a sense of perspective in these moments. The therapist's words and manner must clearly communicate the advice to seek medical evaluation while still keeping in mind that most such tissue changes have a benign cause.

For example:

"Mary, have you felt this area in the upper part of your breast? There's something lumpy right here close to your armpit. It's quite possible that it has been like this before, but this is the first time I've noticed it. It is common for women to have changes taking place in their breasts at menopause, so it could be a variety of things. Has your doctor mentioned it? No? I think you should get your doctor to take a look. It's always best to stay on the safe side. Just keep in mind that almost all of the things that women find and get checked out in their breasts are benign. I shouldn't work directly on something I am not certain of, so I'll move on now. Let me know what your doctor says - I'll feel more comfortable continuing with our treatment plan once it has been checked."

"Paulina, you have a dense section of tissue under this old biopsy scar. Has it always felt like this, I mean since the surgery? It can be difficult with palpation alone to distinguish how extensive scarring is. You could have something else here, though. It feels like the scar tissue is adjoining something lumpy, maybe a cyst. Since the tissue is fibrous from the scar, everything feels firm. When was your last mammogram? Sounds like you are due for one - why not make an appointment to see your doctor and get it checked out? These things usually turn out to be nothing serious. Since we have talked about doing some aggressive work on the scar, I would personally feel more comfortable having it examined before we proceed. The scar makes it harder for me to feel certain about what is happening in the tissue and I don't want to cause any damage. Let me know what Dr. Mossi says."

"LouLou, I'm feeling something lumpy here in your breast. Is that tender? Yes - that's a good sign. The lumps to worry about are usually not painful. You weren't seeing me then, but didn't you mention that you had mastitis when you were breastfeeding? I wonder if it's possible that you have an abscess. You are 39 - it could be several common benign tissue changes as well. Since you are getting used to your breasts again after pregnancy and breastfeeding, why not get a regular check-up and point this lump out to your doctor? If it is an abscess it could cause tissue damage in your breast. I could also make things worse by putting pressure on it, so I'd like to know for sure what it is, myself."

There is a fine line between wanting to give the client a clear message to get a medical evaluation and unduly alarming her. The key components of good client-therapist interaction in this moment are: staying both warm and calm in manner; including the fact that the large majority of all such findings are benign; expressing your need to feel 100% comfortable with your information before proceeding with the treatment plan; and, where applicable, indicating that she is at an age or life cycle stage where tissue changes might be predicted. You can offer a theory about what might be happening, but never cross the line into diagnosis or make guarantees about the outcome.

Since it is not appropriate for the massage therapist to proceed with local treatment when there is a tissue formation which might be cause for concern, the practitioner can easily reinforce the suggestion to seek medical investigation through not wanting to proceed with the treatment plan until they are both satisfied that they know there is nothing happening in the breast that could be adversely affected by massage.

Referral

Knowing when to refer and how to make a good referral are cornerstone skills for all health care practitioners. Referrals can be made instead of or in addition to working with the client oneself. In the context of breast massage, there are several specific reasons why a practitioner may choose to send someone to another massage therapist. The most common include:

- The practitioner does not feel comfortable with breast massage in general, or with offering breast massage to a specific client or type of client.
- The practitioner has cultural or religious grounds for not offering breast massage.
- The practitioner cannot achieve professional neutrality.
- The practitioner is male and the client is more comfortable seeing a female therapist for breast massage.
- The practitioner does not have sufficient training in breast massage, or does not feel competent to work with the type of case the client presents.
- The client might benefit from a different style or approach to the treatment.
- The client would like to be able to receive breast massage in a different area or at a different location.

Researching and providing good referrals is a responsibility of being a health professional. With breast massage, there is the increased challenge of determining which massage therapists offer breast treatment and ensuring that they do so in a framework which will be trustworthy and safe for the client.

Additionally, the massage therapist will want to have on hand a referral list of medical doctors and psychotherapists. These are important resources for breast massage clients who need assistance with breast tissue evaluation or an effective support system to address particular physical or psychoemotional health needs in relation to breast treatment. As well, there are always clients who need second opinions or who are looking for new physicians or psychotherapists. Some mastectomy clients are also interested in finding physiotherapists with whom they can feel comfortable while working on their post-surgical needs.

When making a referral for breast massage, especially in the circumstance where the referring massage therapist is not willing to provide the treatment, it is very important not to imply any judgement of the client or the client's choice to seek out breast massage. The practitioner's management of the situation must be forthright and open, clearly assuming responsibility for not feeling comfortable or for having a specific personal reason for not providing breast massage. The female client in this type of dialogue can be susceptible to all-too-familiar feelings of guilt or inadequacy, so the massage therapist's handling of the conversation needs to consciously avoid any message that might cause or reinforce such feelings.

It is always important to give good thought to matching the client's needs and the style and expertise of the practitioner being referred to, and wherever possible to provide at least two different options.

Becoming More Comfortable as a Practitioner

In retrospect, some clients seem to have been sent to us as gifts. In the mid 80's, about a year after I graduated from massage school, I met Isabel. I was practising in a naturopathic clinic located in an area with a large number of residents of European descent. Isabel was Hungarian. She was 56 at the time and I remember her as a warm feisty woman with a 'full figure.' She was very conscious of being at risk for breast cancer. There were some cases in her family and in her friendship group. She was a strong believer in massage therapy and aware of lymphatic drainage. She spoke to me about breast massage several times. I put her off. I had had one class in school on breast treatment - it was not a solid memory - and although I had felt pretty comfortable in my close-knit class, giving Isabel breast massage didn't feel quite the same. Finally Isabel said to me in comical exasperation and with her wonderful accent: "Debra! I have asked you five times to give me breast massage. You know how to do it and still you don't. You think I will forget about it, right? Well I won't! What can be so hard? I don't mind if you poke me once or twice. What is the matter with you Canadians?" So, I was pretty much behind the eight ball and Isabel began to receive her breast massages. Within six months I was giving her entire extended circle of family and friends breast treatments and had all the practice any massage therapist could ask for. One day I realized I felt completely at ease giving breast massage.

Breast massage has acquired an aura or expectation of being difficult and intricate treatment, but once the practitioner is trained and feels at ease, it is really quite straightforward. The difficulty is definitely not in the techniques, which are simple modifications of familiar massage methods. While there are some massage therapists who have objections to massage therapy for immutable personal or cultural reasons, many simply do not feel ready, or are not confident of doing it properly.

Training programs which offer breast massage are often not entirely comfortable doing so, and as a result provide partial, guarded, or overly quick coverage. One of the most important pieces of feedback we have received from students at our school is that they cannot master their personal lack of ease as well as the techniques and interactions of breast massage in one class session. There seem to be at minimum four steps in learning how to comfortably and effectively do breast massage:

- attaining a level of comfort with simply being in the situation
- addressing and coming to one's own conclusions about the personal/ethical/social/political dilemmas that breast massage can pose for individuals and for massage therapists
- having sufficient hands-on practice
- achieving a sense of ease with the communication skills, interactions and dialogues, and therapeutic relationship scenarios which are inherent to providing breast massage

For some, the challenges can be quite intense, and may require various types of personal and professional support. As has been discussed in previous sections, each massage therapist must assume responsibility for, at minimum, exploring and clearly identifying the nature of and reasons for a strong avoidance, discomfort, or objection reaction. Even if he or she ultimately decides not to offer breast massage, following through on such an exploration will bring the practitioner to a place of awareness and acceptance of his or her personal circumstance and decision, and will help prevent the imparting of confusing or potentially damaging messages to clients.

Once a massage therapy student or practitioner has consciously decided in favour of offering breast massage, has had a basic initiation to the experience of working with breasts, and has received some technical and hands-on instruction, the next step is to practise. This may seem like an obvious statement, but the reality is that most practitioners do not attain enough comfort during their training to feel able to provide breast treatment to their clients. If breast massage is encountered in school as a mandatory learning experience, it may not be followed up with enough practise to ensure that the practitioner feels ready when a client subsequently needs or requests breast work. And, of course, many massage therapists receive no breast massage instruction during their undergraduate education and learn the skills in short advanced training intensives.

It is not a good idea, and is somewhat unsafe in many cases, to 'practise' breast massage with clients who are not aware that you are learning. Family members and friends may be willing to offer opportunities to try out the techniques in a 'forgiving' environment. This kind of help makes it possible for a learner to acquire an amount of experience consistent with achieving hands-on facility. The best situation, perhaps in addition to working with accommodating lay people, is to set up exchanges with a fellow student or colleague, or to find an experienced therapist or breast massage client who is willing to receive breast treatments from you and offer suggestions and feedback. A knowledgeable person like this will have an awareness of the therapeutic relationship skills and boundaries required when offering breast massage, and can help ensure that you have them in place. Massage therapists who are not regularly providing breast treatment, or who feel 'rusty' and are anticipating that they will be asked for or offering breast massage in the near future, can set up this type of practise situation to help them regain the comfort and facility they need.

Even a practitioner who is experienced and familiar with the routines of client-therapist interaction can feel awkward and uncomfortable talking to clients about breast massage. Gaining practise in the handling of these conversations is also needed, both for personal ease and for a better feeling of protection given the societal context and pressures involved.

What follows are some role play scenarios which may help. These are good to practise from both role positions and with varied 'subjects', ideally some of whom are massage colleagues and some not. This will help you get reactions to your approach from different viewpoints. They are exercises which were developed by Pam Fitch, a friend and colleague, for a breast massage advanced training workshop we have designed together. Use them to practise the dialogues related to breast massage, and also to 'remember' the client experience and point of view.

Role Play Scenario #1

Client Maryann has had painful breasts since entering menopause. She has heard that breast massage can help and is very interested in pursuing it. She would like more information first and an opportunity to talk it over with her massage therapist, Joan, whom she likes and trusts. Joan has not given a breast massage since school and is reluctant to offer it now. She has been evading Maryann's gentle attempts to broach the subject and Maryann has begun pushing harder. How does Joan resolve her personal and professional feelings regarding breast massage and how does she respond to Maryann's direct request?

Role Play Scenario #2

Katerina has been a massage therapist for 5 years. In the past year, four of her clients have been diagnosed with breast cancer. Katerina receives breast massage herself on a regular basis from a massage school classmate, but for some reason has not offered it to her clients. A new client, Dana, is scheduled for this morning, having been referred by her physician post-lumpectomy for stress. Katerina treats Dana, but is strongly aware that she is choosing not to provide breast massage care that could give Dana relief of some fairly intense pain and congestion in the affected breast. She also knows that breast massage could help the quality of Dana's developing scar tissue. She decides it is time for her to begin offering breast massage and plans to speak to Dana soon. Dana, for her part, is fearful and reluctant to have her breast touched. How do these women talk with each other about breast massage? How does Katerina prepare herself to provide good quality care to her clients?

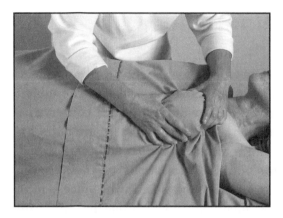

Figure 27. Breast massage through the sheet.

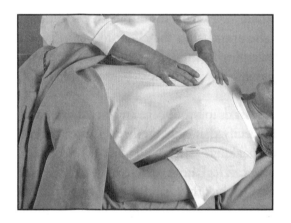

Figure 28. The client is wearing a light cotton T-shirt.

Breast massage through the sheet or a T-shirt can be quite workable for the client who chooses not to have her breasts undraped for treatment. It should be noted that working with a fabric-covered breast can make it more difficult to be accurate in avoiding the nipple, so extra care must be taken. Nipple stimulation can also be the accidental result if the fabric is pulled down and across the anterior breast during the massage therapist's work. When working with a covered breast, the massage therapist needs to be conscious of pushing the fabric inward and slightly upward rather than 'flattening' it and pulling it back and forth over the breast.

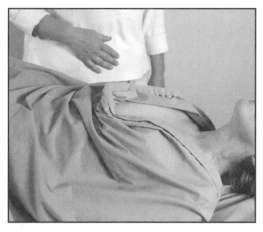
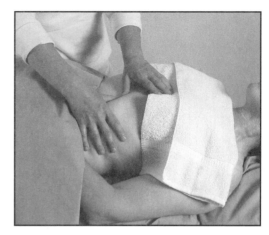

Figure 29   *Figure 30*

When a client is not comfortable having her breasts undraped, the massage therapist can use draping techniques like the ones illustrated in Figures 29 and 30 in order to get good access to the tissues and attachments in the immediate vicinity of the breasts.

Figures 31 and 32 demonstrate a stable sheet design for undraping one breast. This arrangement rarely glides out of place. In Figure 31 the sheet is tucked under the client's side and in Figure 32 it is not. Some clients like the snug, secure feeling of a well-tucked sheet; others find it tight and confining.

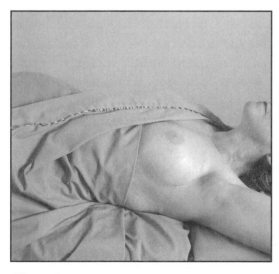
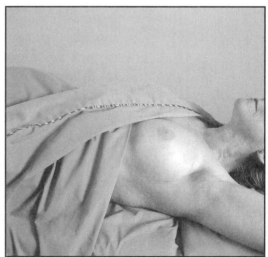

Figure 31   *Figure 32*

Specific Breast Massage Guidelines

As has already been said, the standard general rules and guidelines governing massage therapy apply to breast massage, but perhaps more stringently. This statement is particularly true with respect to therapeutic relationship requirements about communication and consent.

What follows is a summarized list of guidelines applied specifically to breast treatment:

1. Communication, Trust, Consent

- The client responds best to openness, trustworthiness, and common sense in the practitioner. These qualities allow her to form an opinion about the therapeutic relationship environment in which she would be consenting to receive breast massage.

- Most clients need time to consider breast massage. This can include: having informational materials to take home; knowing about her options within the treatment protocol and taking time to think about her reactions and requirements; being given names of clients willing to receive calls from someone considering having breast massage; and having access to as much dialogue with her massage therapist as she needs to feel comfortable.

- The male massage therapist should always offer to refer the client to a female practitioner for breast massage and should have available a list of suitable referrals.

- Breast massage should not proceed until good communication and client-therapist trust is established and the parties have been able to achieve a mutual level of comfort with respect to the proposed treatment plan.

- The consent dialogue must include discussion of the possibility that breast massage may induce emotional reactions or invoke painful memories. The client needs to consider how comfortable she is with this possibility and whether she has an adequate support system in place should she need assistance to deal with reactions like this.

- Breast massage cannot automatically be included in other massage therapy protocols. It is a type of treatment which must be consented to separately and specifically.

- Consent for breast massage must be renewed before each session. The client must clearly understand that she has the right at any time to state a preference, alter or discontinue the treatment plan, or choose not to have breast treatment on a given day.

2. Guidelines for the Therapist

- The massage therapist has the right to decide not to offer breast massage to a particular client, type of client, or at all.

- The massage therapist who cannot achieve good boundaries or professional neutrality must self disqualify from providing breast massage, in general, or in the case of any client who evokes such concerns.

- The practitioner's choice not to offer breast massage must always be communicated in a manner that does not shame or judge the client for seeking out breast treatment.

- Regardless of the specific indications in a client's case, breast massage should always be given in the spirit of aspiring to enhance a woman's positive relationship to her breasts and commitment to breast health care.

- The conscientious massage therapist assumes responsibility for helping a client familiarize herself with her breast tissues, for supporting regular breast medical evaluation and self examination, and for encouraging breast self massage.

- The massage therapist must not sexualize the breast massage situation. This includes refraining from using language about breasts or making statements about a client's breasts which create a sexual inference. The therapist must avoid touching or in other ways stimulating the nipples. Any indication from a client that she finds the breast treatment arousing does not change the practitioner's responsibilities in these respects.

- The practitioner must make every attempt to self monitor for personal issues and reactions which might jeopardize the integrity of the therapeutic relationship. He or she must also seek to be 'present' and focused during breast treatment to avoid creating an atmosphere which could be misinterpreted. Overly sensitive or solicitous behaviour is also avoided.

- The practitioner must seek out training adequate to the demands of his or her practice. In the breast massage context this could include both technical skills training and therapeutic relationship skill-building. It may also include advanced education in handling more complex psychoemotional situations.

3. Technical Guidelines

- Breast massage techniques should be designed to enhance and support lymphatic drainage, the predominant drainage system of the breast, incorporating the understanding that most lymph flow in the breast is anterior to posterior.

- Breast treatment will be most effective when it is preceded by relaxation of surrounding musculature which can compress on its neural and circulatory supplies, in particular pectoralis major.

- Manual techniques should not overstress or overstretch the supporting membrane structure of the breast.

- Draping procedures will always conform to the client's wishes.

- It is especially important that the client feels warm, comfortable, and physically secure for breast work.

- The massage therapist needs to keep in mind that painful breasts, recent surgery or trauma, some breast conditions, and the presence of breast implants may necessitate positioning adaptations during general massage therapy. Prone position, and at times sidelying, may be too uncomfortable to be utilized.

4. Special Considerations

- Standard post-surgical guidelines apply when treating a client who has recently had a breast procedure. These include: observation for complications like thrombosis, particular attention to hygiene in the vicinity of the incision, caution about compressing or displacing drainage tubes, caution during positioning and turning of the client, application of hydrotherapy which is consistent with tissue tolerances and the efficacy of local circulatory channels, and avoidance of overly early stressing of the incision site and repairing tissues by manual techniques or passive movements.

- If the client has or has had breast cancer, the massage therapist needs to be familiar with risks, adaptations, and guidelines pertaining to massage therapy for the person with cancer.* This important subject involves a number of aspects which require the massage practitioner's attention. Breast cancer does not have specific or unique features in this respect; however, it is important for the practitioner to be knowledgeable about and feel comfortable with the blend of breast massage and cancer-related considerations.

- For clients with mastectomies, breasts which have been removed, like other 'phantom' parts, often have an energetic presence for the woman. The tissue area should be approached with the sensitivity and respect accorded to breasts.

- Massage therapists should have an awareness of stability and obsolescence concerns related to breast implants.

* The reader may wish to reference Curties, D. 'Massage Therapy and Cancer', Curties-Overzet Publications, 1998.

HOW TO DO BREAST MASSAGE

Breast Massage Techniques

The techniques of breast massage are not in any way complex. They are largely modifications of common petrissage strokes adapted to the size and shape of the breast. Once a practitioner feels comfortable with the idea of working with breasts and with the inherent client-therapist relationship requirements, mastery of the technical skills is quite simple and straightforward.

There are four key elements to keep in mind when designing a hands-on protocol for breast treatment:

1. There are no dense structures like muscles present in the breast. Routine massage of breasts without scars is geared to enhancement of circulation and drainage - it does not usually involve firm pressure or 'stripping' types of techniques. Overly aggressive work may damage the membranous supporting tissues of the breast.

2. Anatomically, breast circulation channels and pain pathways can be strongly affected by muscular and postural factors in neighbouring structures. Breast massage will be most effective once such structures, especially pectoralis major, have been treated and relaxed.

3. Breast work must prioritize lymphatic drainage. This includes stimulating lymphatic clearance channels and nodes before specific breast tissue work is done, recognizing the need to mobilize the tissues 'up and off' the retromammary space during treatment, and incorporating the knowledge that the majority of lymph drainage travels posteriorly through the breast before exiting into its external drainage channels.

4. Hands-on work must consciously avoid touching the nipple.

The techniques on these pages are offered as a framework or set of suggestions. There is ample room for individual practitioners to make modifications and to incorporate ideas or techniques they may have picked up from other types of training. Any techniques which are consistent with the considerations and principles discussed in previous sections will be appropriate for inclusion in breast treatment protocols.

Preliminary Stimulation of Lymphatic Channels

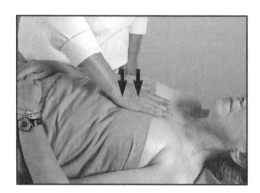

Figure 33

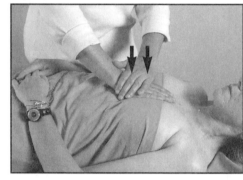

Figure 34

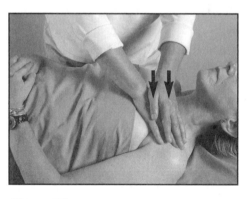

Figure 35

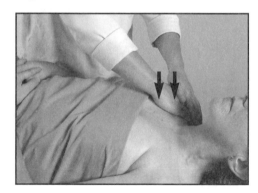

Figure 36

Figures 33-36 show the practitioner gently 'pumping' the sternum and clavicles to stimulate lymph flow and activity in the regional lymph nodes. This work assists the efficiency of lymphatic drainage at the beginning of the breast treatment. Massage therapists with specific lymphatic drainage training will have the advantage of being able to incorporate more advanced types of techniques. Figures 33 and 34 demonstrate sternal 'pumping' and Figures 35 and 36 show clavicular 'pumping'.

Relaxation of Neighbouring Muscles

Pectoralis Major: Figures 37 through 46 illustrate a sequence of techniques which address pectoralis major and its various attachment sites.

Figure 37
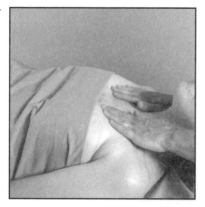

Figure 38
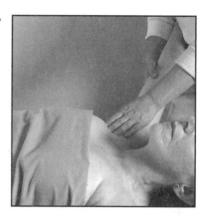

Figure 39
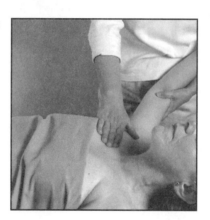

Figure 40
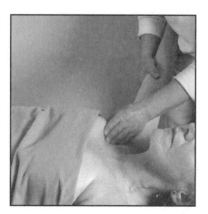

Figure 41
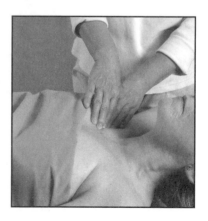

Figure 42

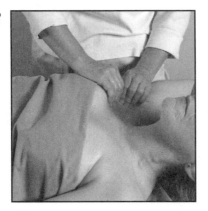

Figure 43

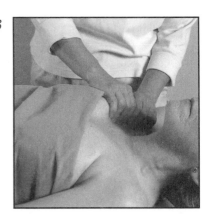

Figure 44

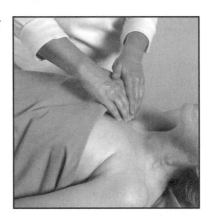

Figure 45

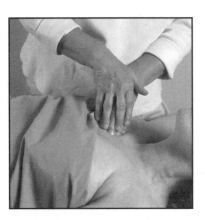

Figure 46

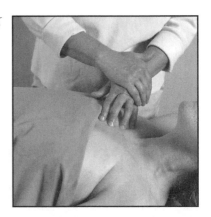

Figure 47

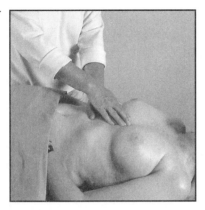

Figure 48

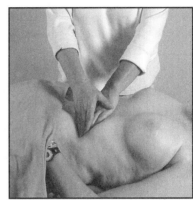

Other Muscles:

Figures 47 and 48 show specific work at the subcostal angle and along the distal ribcage to address rectus abdominis attachments. Figures 49 through 51 show techniques directed at the intercostal muscles, and to some extent, serratus anterior.

Figure 49

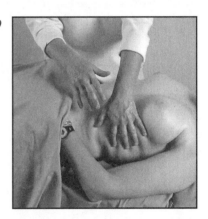

Figure 50

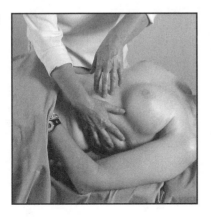

Figure 51

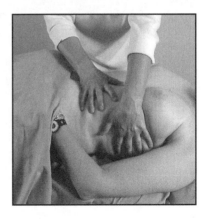

Beginning the Breast Treatment

Effleurage of the breasts can be approached from a superior direction, as illustrated in Figures 52 through 55 below...

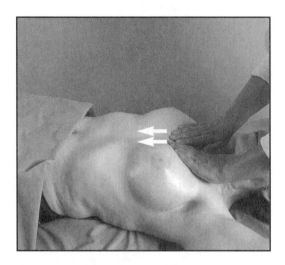

Figure 52

Figure 53

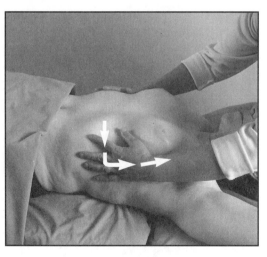

Figure 54

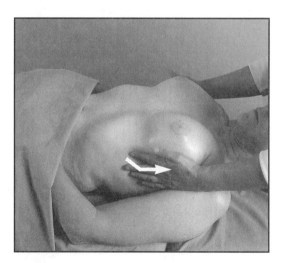

Figure 55

... or with the massage therapist standing beside the client, as in Figures 56 through 60.

Figure 56

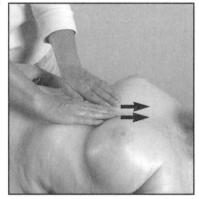

Figure 57

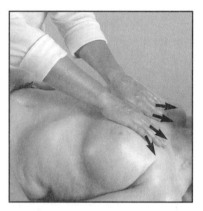

Figure 58

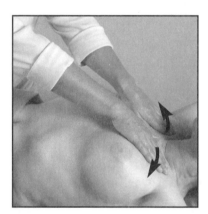

Figure 59

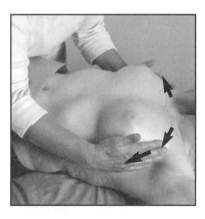

Figure 60

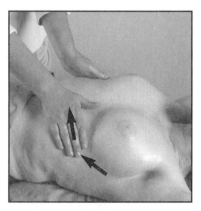

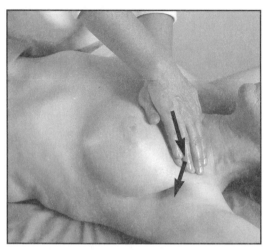

Figure 61

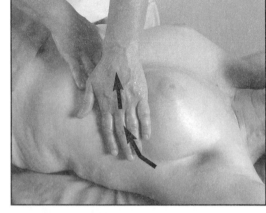

Figure 62

The massage therapist can also effleurage around one breast at a time. This may be done after an effleurage sequence involving both breasts. When the choice of draping involves uncovering one breast at a time, the style of effleurage shown in Figures 61 through 63 is most suitable.

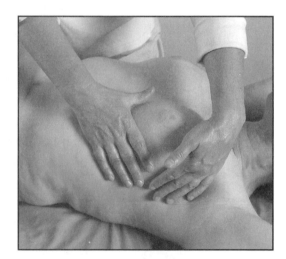

Figure 63

Petrissage Strokes

As a natural continuation of the effleurage around each breast, the practitioner can next deepen the hand pressure and make it more specific. As is illustrated in Figures 64 to 66, this will transition the treatment into petrissage. The emphasis shifts to mobilizing the breast tissue, including beginning to incorporate some anterior 'lift'.

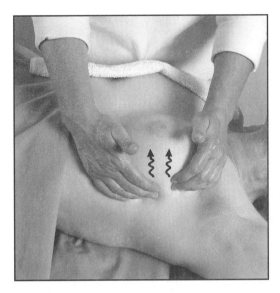

Figure 64

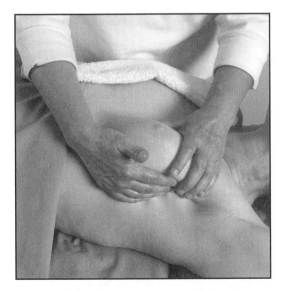

Figure 65

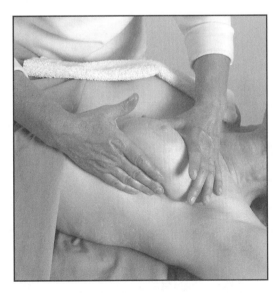

Figure 66

Next, with the therapist still using a full-handed approach, the breast tissue is moved back and forth. Notice in Figures 67 to 70 that the practitioner's hands shift position in order to address the tissue from different angles.

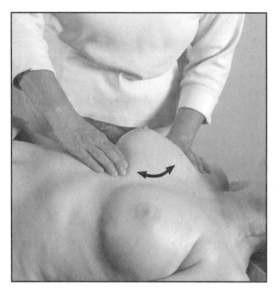

Figure 67

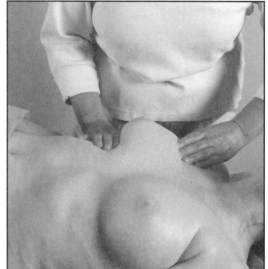

Figure 68

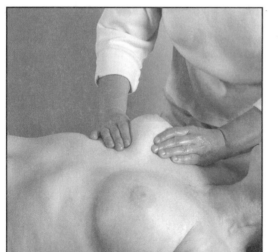

Figure 69

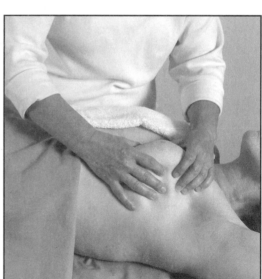

Figure 70

In Figures 71-74, the massage therapist's fingers transition to more specific strokes. This practitioner is right-handed - observe the kneading action she begins to incorporate with her right hand while continuing to shift her hand positions in the same manner as before.

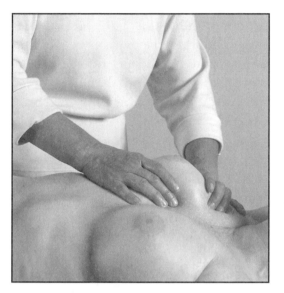

Figure 71

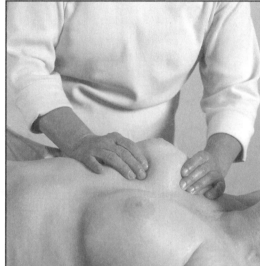

Figure 72

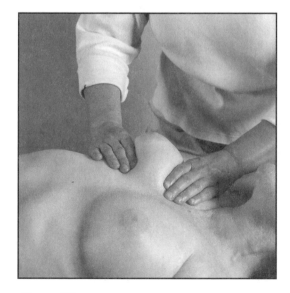

Figure 73

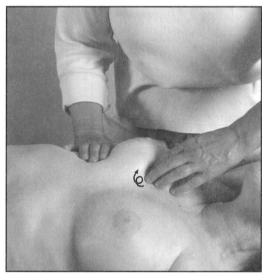

Figure 74

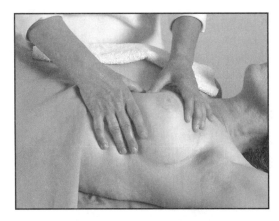

Figure 75

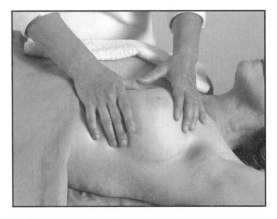

Figure 76

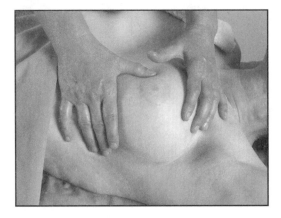

Figure 77

Figures 75 through 77 illustrate alternate thumb kneading. This stroke is usually performed in lines along the breast tissue. Always treating the medial side of the breast opposite, the practitioner would move to the other side of the table in order to work on the lateral tissue of the breast currently being treated. Note that the massage therapist has put a towel over the client's right breast because she is leaning over it while she does this kneading. Notice also the position of her fingers - she is holding her hands in such a way that she avoids 'drifting' over the nipple.

Working from the outside to the centre of the breast is consistent with mobilizing both the venous and lymphatic drainage to their subareolar plexi.

The practitioner can choose to add or substitute circular fingertip kneading (not demonstrated) or other similar specific strokes as he or she prefers. This type of stroke is useful in mobilizing the more superficial tissues and their drainage, but should not be a large percentage of the treatment.

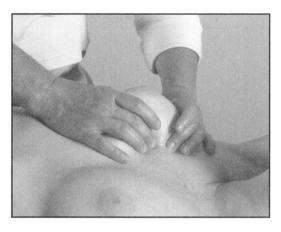

Figure 78

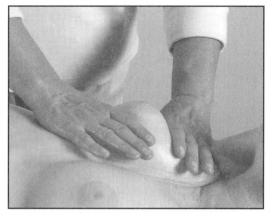

Figure 79

Figures 78 through 80 demonstrate one of the most important sequences of the treatment. In Figures 78 and 79, the breast is alternately lifted and compressed to create a 'pumping' action on the retromammary space. The breast is also 'jiggled' with a fine shaking action in which it is rapidly moved to and fro with the therapist's hands assuming various stable positions around its outer aspect (Figure 80). These strokes can be done in any sequence to achieve completeness in mobilizing the breast tissues.

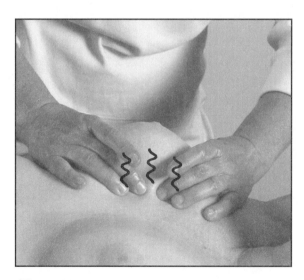

Figure 80

To finish the breast massage, the practitioner can choose his or her preferred effleurage approach(es).

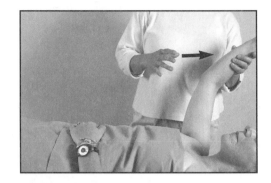

Figure 83

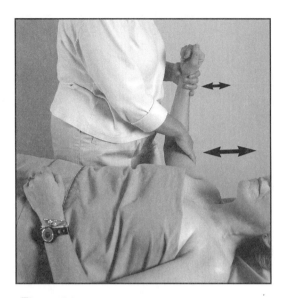

Figure 81

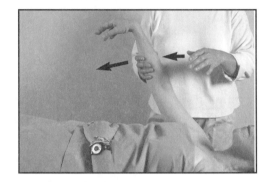

Figure 84

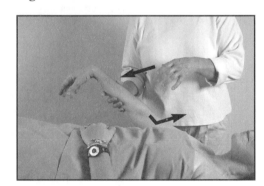

Figure 85

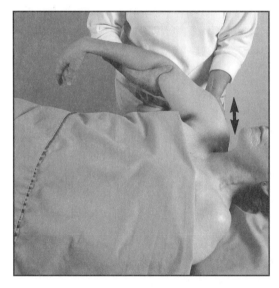

Figure 82

Figures 81 through 85 show the massage therapist mobilizing the client's shoulder. Done bilaterally, this shoulder mobilization aids in relaxing musculature and adds to the stimulation of blood and lymph flow related to the breast. These techniques, or similar ones preferred by the practitioner, can be utilized at the beginning and/or end of the treatment, or interspersed throughout.

Self Massage for Clients

On this page and its reverse are photographs of self massage techniques for clients to use at home. Technique is not the most important thing - these illustrations show easy ways to massage all the parts of the breast and to finish with strokes that encourage drainage.

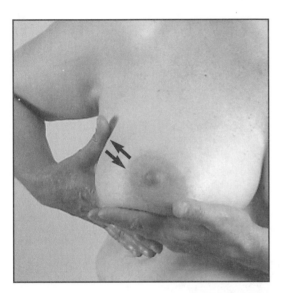
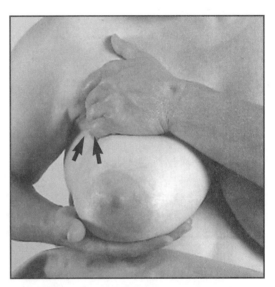
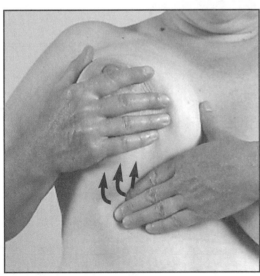
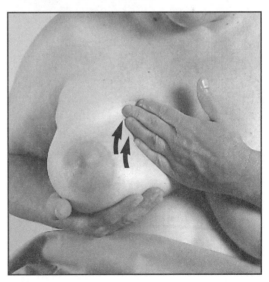

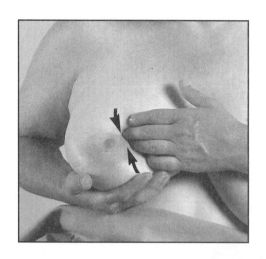

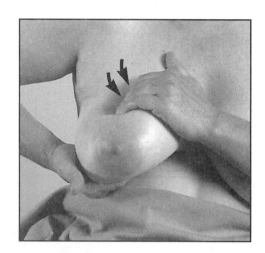

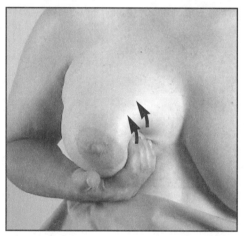

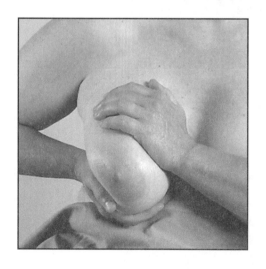

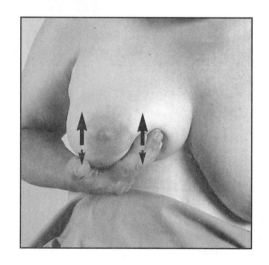

Breast Massage During Pregnancy and Breastfeeding

Many women choose to have breast massage during pregnancy and lactation, even if they would not ordinarily be so inclined. In fact, it is during these reproductive cycles that women are often introduced to the benefits of breast treatment.

The pregnant/breastfeeding woman experiences her breasts in new and different ways. They are perceived more clearly as 'working' body parts. There is a focus on managing breast tissue changes so that the pregnant woman can maximize her physical comfort and sense of wellbeing, and so that the mother and her infant can enjoy the benefits of successful nursing. As has been outlined in an earlier section, pregnant women usually experience some degree of breast discomfort, typically consisting of marked tenderness in months 2 through 4 and heaviness and aching in the last trimester. Nursing mothers routinely report breast congestion and pain, especially early and late in the breastfeeding period. Although there are variations in the degree to which women experience these symptoms, it is rare for them to be completely absent. The high priority most mothers place on successful breastfeeding tends to create a strong awareness of breast health and a much higher than usual priority on finding needed assistance and symptom relief.

Breast massage for the client who is pregnant or breastfeeding does not have significantly different features from a technical point of view. In other words, there is no 'pregnancy' or 'lactating' treatment for breasts. Some specific considerations can be outlined as follows:

1. Emotional Factors

The hormonal fluctuations in the pregnant or breastfeeding woman's body, and the significance of this time in her life and that of her family, can add to the intensity of psychoemotional reactions she may have to receiving breast massage.

2. Use of Sidelying Position

The massage therapist needs to be adaptable about doing breast treatment in sidelying position. Most clients have difficulty breathing and generally feel uncomfortable lying supine in later pregnancy. It is also not an ideal position for the client or for the fetus because it tends to compress the baby onto her low back and large blood vessels. The massage practitioner needs to be versatile about position adaptations, anyway. Breast massage clients may at times need to be placed in sidelying for reasons unrelated to pregnancy. Figures 86-88 illustrate breast massage in sidelying position. Standing behind the client seems to give the best tissue access and orientation for the therapist's hands.

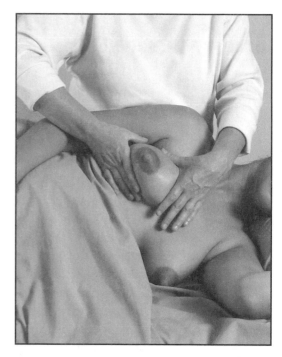

Figure 86

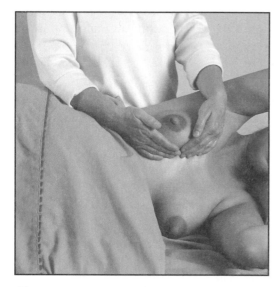

Figure 87

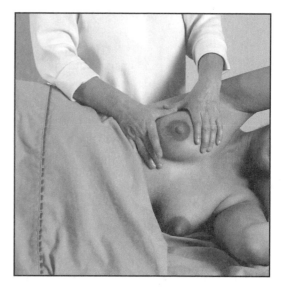

Figure 88

3. Use of the Cold Figure 8 Wrap

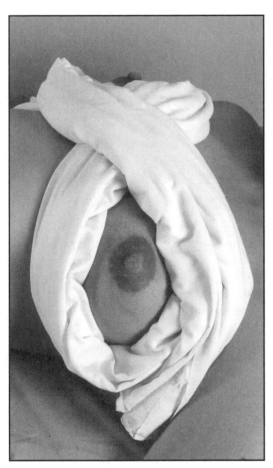

Figure 89

A percentage of women experience breast tenderness in early pregnancy and immediately postpartum to the point of not wanting to have their breasts touched at all. With or without doing breast massage, the practitioner can often achieve excellent symptom relief with cold wrap treatments.

A sheet (twin size is best) is soaked in cold water - ice water as long as the client does not object. The sheet must be well wrung out before placement. If water is not available and a refrigerator is, the sheet can be placed dry in the freezer in advance.

Figure 89 shows the way the sheet is wrapped around the client's breasts. When the sheet warms up it can be resoaked in the cold water and re-applied.

This same application can be used for other reasons as well, for example as a hot modality before scar work, or as a contrast modality for congestion or chronic edema.

4. Hygiene Concerns

It is important for the massage therapist to remember that the lactating mother's breasts are susceptible to mastitis. The reader may want to refer to the prior section on this subject. The nursing baby can cause small skin lesions to form in the vicinity of the nipple and areola, which may or may not be visible, and common bacteria can use these to gain access to the breast tissues. Despite not touching the nipple directly, the practitioner must recognize the need for particular attention to the hygienic condition of his or her hands, the lubricant used, and hydrotherapy application materials.

5. Expression of Milk

It is very likely that massaging lactating breasts will cause them to express milk, as is illustrated in Figure 90. There is absolutely no reason to be concerned or embarrassed about this. In fact, it may happen even without the manual stimulation of massage techniques, but just from lying supine, changing position, or from the breasts becoming full. If the baby is nearby, hearing it cry can also cause its mother's breasts to release milk.

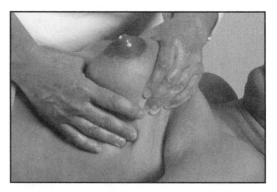

Figure 90

6. Musculoskeletal Factors Can Cause Discomfort for the Breastfeeding Mother

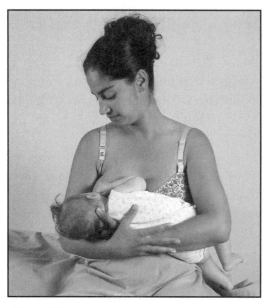

Figure 91

Figure 91 illustrates the position typically used by the nursing mother. On close observation, it is easy to pinpoint the musculoskeletal stresses this position can cause, especially as the baby gets heavier. In addition to common complaints the woman may have, for example headaches, mid-back pain, thoracic outlet syndrome, and so on, postural and muscular overuse stresses may contribute to pain and circulatory congestion in her breasts.

The muscles in greatest need of attention are usually the scalenes, levator scapulae, trapezius, and all the posterior cervical muscles. Pectoralis major and minor are generally shortened and tight.

As well, there are interrelated postural stresses which affect the nursing mother's whole body. It is noteworthy that many women particularly notice their hip flexors (psoas) and calf muscles becoming sore and short from long sitting and from propping their toes to help hold the baby up into position. This body configuration also tends to contribute to upper body hyperkyphotic patterns.

Post-Surgical Breast Massage and Techniques for Scar Work

Common Breast Surgical Procedures

The Figures which follow illustrate the surgical procedures most commonly used on breasts. This information is presented in order to demonstrate the types of tissue intervention involved and the scars which would be expected to result.

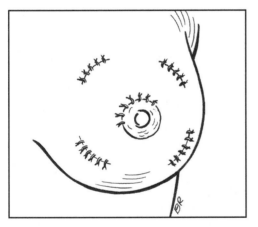

Figure 92 shows the types of incisions used for biopsies or removal of small lesions, for example cysts.

Figure 92

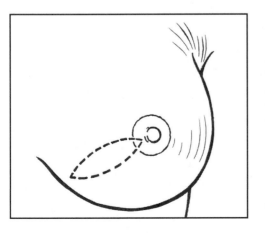

Figure 93 illustrates the surgical opening needed to remove a ductal or lobar segment of tissue. The resulting scar can span most of the breast radius.

Figure 93

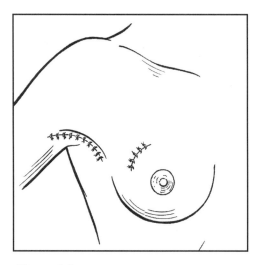

Figure 94

Figure 94 represents the incision pattern seen when a woman has a biopsy or lumpectomy and axillary lymph node exploration. In the past, excavation for lymph nodes was often very extensive. Sampling is more common now; in fact, it was recently discovered that one of the axillary system nodes is situated in such a way in the lymph channels that whether or not it contains cancer cells is probably predictive of spread to others. This node is being referred to as the 'sentinel node'. Smaller and smaller incisions in the axilla are likely in future as the trend toward removal of a limited number of specific nodes for evaluation becomes established as normal practice.

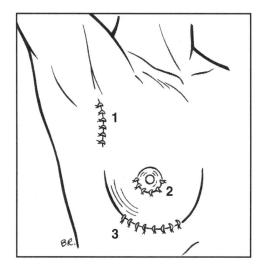

Figure 95

Figure 95 shows the three options for surgical incisions used in placement of breast implants:

1. axillary
2. periareolar
3. inframammary

Mastectomy

Mastectomy is removal of the breast, typically because of cancer. In the past, it was fairly routine to remove sections of pectoralis major and all or most of the regional lymph nodes. Neither of these is as common an occurrence now.

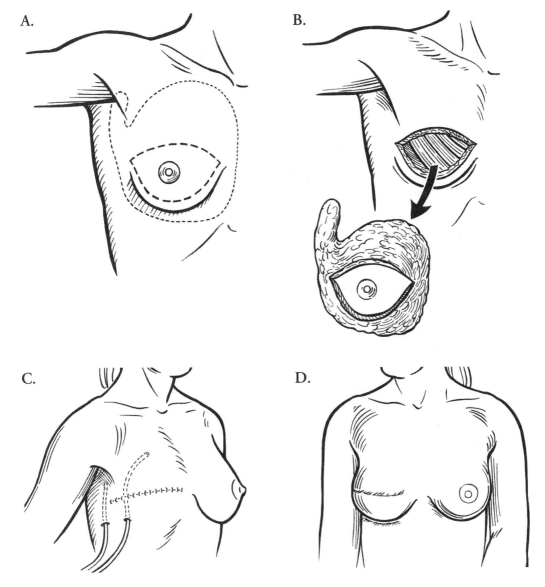

Figure 96

Figure 96. This Figure follows the process of a standard procedure mastectomy through to subsequent placement of an implant. In A. the incision zone is outlined; B. illustrates removal of the breast tissue; C. shows the surgical site with placement of drainage tubes; and in D. an implant has been placed via an inframammary incision. The nipple is usually added 6-8 weeks later, via skin flap transplant or tattooing, once the tissue has stabilized and the post-surgical edema has subsided.

Figure 96 shows the incision usually used for mastectomy. Some surgeons argue that a diagonal cut across the breast with the top end pointing toward the axilla leaves a scar which is more amenable to implant placement and is less likely to be seen with low cut clothing like bathing suits.

Mastectomy is obviously an emotionally difficult experience for most women. While many surgeons prefer to wait for the tissue to stabilize and to assess the results of the surgery, it has been found that women are often more comfortable with the process if a reconstruction procedure is done at the same time as the mastectomy.

Breast Augmentation

Augmentation procedures are performed for three main reasons:

1. To increase the size of a woman's breasts because she perceives them as too small (cosmetic augmentation). 75-80% of breast enlargement is done for this reason[106].

2. To correct breast asymmetry or a loss of breast tissue due to trauma or other occurrence.

3. As a reconstruction procedure following mastectomy.

Augmentation is most frequently done with implants. It is common for the surgeon to use a tissue expander before implantation, especially if the breast is very small or has been removed. The expander is an inflatable device which is inserted under the skin and subcutaneous tissue and progressively filled with saline over a period of up to three months. The saline solution is injected through a small subcutaneous valve. The goal is to stretch the tissue to 30% beyond the ultimate desired size in order to accommodate for tissue retraction and to reduce the probability of problematic capsular contractures. The expander is removed at the time of the augmentation procedure.

Myocutaneous Flaps

Myocutaneous flap procedures have been steadily gaining acceptance since they came into use in the 1970's. In this type of procedure breasts are enlarged or reconstructed using transplanted tissue from the woman's own body. The indications for a myocutaneous flap over an implant are:

1. The woman prefers not to use implants because of the concerns that have arisen about them.

2. The woman is having the procedure following explantation.

3. Women who have had radiation therapy may not have the quality or quantity of usable skin needed to cover an implant, and therefore benefit from a procedure which imports tissue to the site.

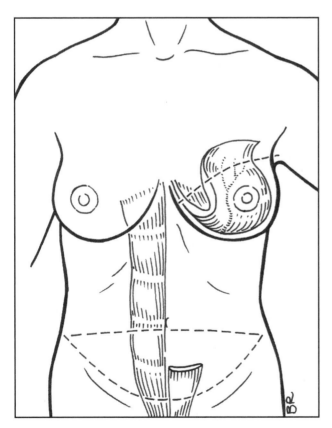

Figure 97

Figure 97 shows the most commonly performed myocutaneous flap operation. It is called the transverse rectus abdominis myocutaneous (TRAM) procedure. In this illustration the transplanted section of rectus abdominis is on the same side as the reconstruction; it is increasingly common for the contralateral side of the muscle to be used. In either case, the section of muscle is passed up to the site under the skin and subcutaneous tissue of the abdominal wall. An attempt is made to preserve the transplanted tissue's nerve and blood supply. The access needed to move the muscle transplant in this way requires the large abdominal incision shown.

Another version of this procedure involves cutting away a section of the abdominal wall and rectus abdominis muscle, using the same incision pattern given in Figure 97, and moving it as a 'free' flap into position to shape a breast. This procedure has a somewhat higher transplant failure rate, but is preferable if the woman lacks viable skin.

The TRAM procedures have good patient satisfaction ratings. Many women like the 'tummy tuck' aspect. Significant abdominal muscle insufficiency is reported in a small percentage of cases - one study reports 2 cases out of 50[107].

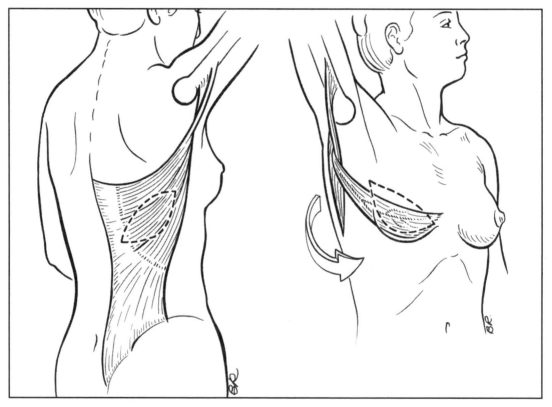

Figure 98

Figure 98 illustrates the second type of myocutaneous flap procedure, the latissimus dorsi flap. A section of latissimus dorsi is stripped and moved through the axilla, usually with an attached pedicle of tissue which helps preserve its neural and blood supply, to augment or reconstruct the ipsilateral breast.

An implant may be placed under the transplanted flap, or a section of attached fat may be moved with the transplanted muscle in order to construct a larger breast.

The latissimus dorsi flap is recommended if the woman wants to become pregnant in the future. As well, some women prefer the scar on the back to the large abdominal one from the TRAM operations. It is also the preferred autologous tissue procedure for bilateral placements.

Women report few muscle problems as a result of the latissimus dorsi transplant. They may tire more easily with overhead actions and feel some loss of strength with maximal activities like the power stroke in swimming.

It is typical for the woman to be uncomfortable lying supine for 2-3 months following this operation, largely because of soreness and skin tightness at the transplant site. Massage therapy can be very helpful in ameliorating these symptoms.

All of the myocutaneous flap procedures are susceptible to hematoma and edema formation. They usually have drains for several days, sometimes as much as two weeks. It is also customary for the nipple to be created or tattooed at a later date, once the tissue has 'normalized' and good matching of the two nipples can be done.

Breast Reduction

Operations to reduce breast size are performed for two main reasons:

1. The woman is unhappy with the size of her breasts because she has difficulty with the type of attention they receive, finding clothes that fit, and so on, and is seeking to improve her body image.
2. The woman is experiencing neck, shoulder, and/or back problems because of the weight of her breasts.

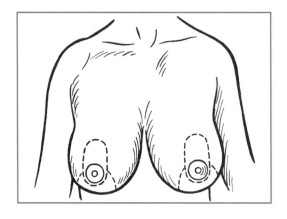

Figure 99 illustrates how the incisions are made, where excess tissue is removed, and the scar pattern that results from breast reduction. This is the widely used procedure, called the Wise Keyhole, after Dr. Robert Wise who developed it in 1956.

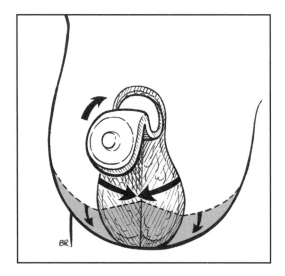

While initially quite painful, this surgery usually resolves well and has a very high patient satisfaction rating. In a study[108] of 328 women, 94.2% rated their procedure as completely or very successful. Pregnancy, aging, and changes in body weight can compromise the symmetry and shape of reduced breasts. Women who had the procedure at 20 or younger express less satisfaction than those who average age 40 at the time the operation is done.

There is some risk that the viability of the nipple may be compromised. Both nipple and lower quadrant breast sensation are usually impaired to some extent, and women who have had this procedure often experience problems with breastfeeding.

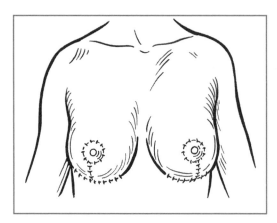

Figure 99

Post-Surgical Breast Massage

Breast surgery is common - surgical procedures are regularly utilized for diagnostic, therapeutic, and cosmetic purposes. In most cases, especially if the woman is otherwise healthy and free of complicating conditions (chemotherapy, diabetes, and steroid use are three examples of factors which may delay or impair recovery), her return to daily life is quite rapid. A significant number of these women, however, have lingering problems with edema, pain, and uncomfortable scar formations which can be esthetically and symptomatically troubling. Although there has been very little research into the efficacy of breast massage in treating post-surgical symptoms, massage practitioners who do this type of work in clinical practice report tremendous improvements in cases involving both recent and old procedures.

The guiding principles for providing post-surgical massage on the breast, or a mastectomy site, are the same as those for other body parts. However, since this is an area of treatment with which massage practitioners have varying degrees of experience, it is useful to summarize them here.

1. Consultation

It is better to consult than to make an error in clinical judgement. If the massage therapist feels uncertain about the viability of a surgical site, or how best to design a compatible massage therapy treatment plan, it is advisable to consult with the client's physician before beginning on-site work. The most likely causes for concern, as will be outlined next, are presence/risk of infection, local circulatory problems, and resilience of the recovering tissues with respect to stressors associated with massage techniques, hydrotherapy, and movement modalities.

There are also considerations in working with clients who have cancer which often require consultation with their medical team members. Information about predicted post-surgical cancer cell activity, implications of tissue losses and lymph node excisions, and healing complications caused by concurrent radiation and chemotherapy are common areas of consultation. The reader wanting more information about treatment planning for the massage therapy client with cancer may wish to read Curties, D., *Massage Therapy and Cancer*, Curties-Overzet Publications, 1998. This body of knowledge cannot be given adequate coverage in this text but is important information for the therapist working with the post-surgical client whose procedure was performed because of breast cancer.

2. Hygienic Concerns

Infection greatly complicates post-surgical tissue healing and can delay or impede recovery. The viability of implants and flaps can also be compromised. Local post-surgical treatment approaches must wait until the incision and any other open tissues are well sealed. Observation for delayed healing, oozing or other indications that the skin surface has not closed, and signs of developing infection are all part of routine clinical practice.

Epitheliarization across a stitched incision is usually complete in 2-3 days. This makes the wound resistant to passage of infective organisms, but it is a fragile surface which can be jeopardized by physical stressors and lubricants like oil. Clients with extensive surgical wounds or causes of delayed healing may not conform to the 2-3 day time frame. If infection does set in, tissue repair is usually considered to begin once it has been resolved. Delays of this nature, along with the tissue irritation organisms can cause, may produce a poorer quality of repair.

The massage therapist must exercise all usual hygienic precautions, and give careful consideration to the hygienic state of any substance (oils/lotions, hydrotherapy application materials, etc.) coming in close contact with the early surgical site.

3. Drains

Some breast procedures involve use of drainage tubes which may be left in place for several days, sometimes longer. These drains impose the following considerations on the massage practitioner:

- They can be a conduit for movement of organisms, so any handling of them should involve proper hygienic precautions.
- They should not be pulled out. While it is unlikely that the massage therapist would do so deliberately, it is easy to tug on drains inadvertently with incautious hands-on work, when securing draping, and during positioning of the client.
- The client should not lie on them for extended periods of time.

4. Concerns About Local Circulation

Surgeons take great pains to avoid circulatory complications, but given the vascular disruption caused by surgical procedures, these problems do from time to time develop:

- **hematoma** - collection of blood seepage in a clotted mass in the tissue which often needs to be evacuated to prevent healing complications
- **thrombosis** - development of a clot-like mass called a thrombus inside an artery or vein; direct or mechanical pressures on thrombi can cause intensification of the thrombosis, leading to tissue death from vessel occlusion, or breaking off of the thrombus and propulsion of the loose structure into the bloodstream as an embolus
- **aneurysm** - bulging of a weakened blood vessel wall; the concern is that it may rupture or promote local thrombus formation
- **ischemia** - reduced blood supply to the surgical site
- **excessive edema** - swelling which is greater than, or lasts longer than would be considered normal; increased pain, reduced tissue nutrition, and promotion of bacterial proliferation can result

The massage therapist's observation of the surgical site should involve alertness for tissue discolouration indicating either blood collection or ischemic states, abnormal tissue temperature in the hot or cool directions, fluid accumulation levels beyond the norm, and any unusual bulging or pulsing of local vessels.

Presence of any of the above circulatory complications contraindicates local massage - the site should be re-evaluated by the physician. The massage therapist can play an important role in making timely referrals which can help get problems addressed quickly.

The massage therapist also needs to exercise judgement about overly early use of manual techniques and hydrotherapy applications which might put too much load on the local circulatory channels.

5. Pain

A few days of intense pain are the norm following most surgical procedures. The pain then usually tapers off over a period of time extending from several additional days to much longer time frames depending on the nature of the operation. Breast procedures are often painful beyond the woman's expectations. The pain can persist in ways that affect her quality of life as she resumes daily activities. This happens in part because breast surgery is done by cutting directly through the structure - breast tissue organization does not provide viable planes or layers for the surgeon to follow. Implant placement, as has been discussed in detail in a previous section, is also commonly quite painful.

Post-surgical pain reflects the amount of tissue and blood vessel damage incurred, as well as some degree of aggravation of local nerves. This aggravation can be the result of injuries incurred during the operation or of irritation or compression from blood or edema. Nerve-related pain may be more persistent than pain from other sources. Injured nerves can cause symptoms for as much as a year while they undergo repair, and permanent nerve damage can create ongoing pain syndromes.

Pain symptoms may reflect increased transmission along nociceptive fibres or may be the result of altered large fibre inputs which ordinarily help to inhibit pain sensation. As well, nerves may be 'stunned' or less active for a period of time post-surgically and begin to create or increase symptom presentation after some delay. For example, the onset of transitory forearm and/or hand pain 4-6 weeks post-surgically is a fairly common occurrence. Procedures closely affecting the nipple or brachial plexus are most likely to cause a predominance of neural symptoms.

Assuming proper precautions are taken in handling the injured tissues, the massage therapist has an array of effective methods for helping the client relieve or reduce pain. It is important to be aware that analgesic medications may impair the client's ability to give accurate feedback.

Excessive or otherwise unusual pain should always be grounds for referral to a physician for further evaluation.

6. Fatigue

Many women experience prolonged fatigue after extensive breast surgery, especially mastectomy. There are probably a combination of physical and emotional reasons for this. It is not uncommon for the massage therapist to encounter clients who cannot comprehend why they persist in feeling tired. It is best to encourage them to get the rest they need and not place expectations on how quickly the fatigue should go away.

7. Sensory Abnormalities

It is quite common for clients to have areas of tissue numbness following breast surgeries, especially the more extensive ones like mastectomy, augmentation, and reduction. Lost or reduced sensation should always cause the massage therapist to exercise greater caution, since the client cannot give routine types of feedback about uncomfortable pressures or temperatures. The practitioner needs to rely more heavily on palpatory skill and tissue observation to ascertain appropriate levels of treatment.

The client may also experience abnormal sensations like paraesthesia ('pins and needles', skin crawling, or similar sensations), dysesthesia (painful paraesthesias like 'hot pokers'), and allodynia (sensory stimuli which ordinarily do not produce pain are doing so). Exaggerated or irritable sensation is also fairly common; in other words, the intensity of a stimulus like pressure or temperature is being experienced as much greater than would be predicted as a normal reaction.

Sensory changes that persist for longer than a year are generally considered to be permanent. The massage therapist should always question a client who has had breast surgery about areas of altered tissue sensation.

8. Tissue Resilience[105]

The following are norms for regeneration and repair of typical incision wounds:

- first 18-24 hours - development of a 'crust'
- first 2-3 days - completion of surface epitheliarization which forms beneath the crust
- 2nd to 7th days - shrinkage and dehydration of the crust leading to eventual shedding
- at 5-7 days - usual time stitches are removed
- beginning after the first 5-6 days and lasting about 60 days - formation and placement of collagen, initially as fragile fibrils which in time mature into fibres with tensile strength; as part of the maturation process collagen fibres also cross-link with each other to create a 'structure'
- on average 3 months, but can be up to a year - time period it takes to maximize the tensile strength of the scar (it only achieves about 80% of the previous tissue strength)

After the first two weeks the scar has about 7% of its ultimate tissue strength; after 3 weeks, 20%; and after 1 month, 50%. Delayed repair can occur for various reasons, the most common of which are:

excessive dryness or wetness of the wound, infection, hematoma, the person's poor nutritional status, oxygen deprivation of the healing tissue (usually ischemic, may be bad bandaging), underlying illnesses or conditions, and premature tension or stress of the wound.

The massage therapist should not begin to apply direct stresses to the site until 10-14 days post-surgically, assuming tissue repair is proceeding in the expected time frame, so that collagen deposition and fibre cross-linking can reach a point where the early scar can withstand appropriate levels of tension. Once this stage has been reached, manual therapy and functional stretching can help optimize the alignment of the fibres in order to reduce pain and help the scar accommodate to customary tissue movements and usages.

In addition to exercising caution with manual techniques and range of motion work, the practitioner needs to be alert to potential overstressing of a recent surgical site during positioning and turning of the client.

9. Post-Mastectomy Edema

Mastectomies can produce extensive edema and often involve placement of drains for several days post-surgically. A 'pad' of swelling may linger at the site, to the extent that it is not uncommon for women to express concern about whether all the breast tissue has been removed.

Lymphatic drainage techniques can be highly effective in normalizing fluid retention post-surgically. Alternating light effleurage and petrissage can also make an effective treatment. Lymph node removal is the usual cause of persistent edema which primarily affects the arm and hand. Fortunately, the trend to remove fewer nodes has helped reduce this problem for many women. If there is permanently impaired lymph clearance through the axillary system of nodes, the massage therapist can play an important role in helping to mobilize drainage toward the internal mammary system. If the scar is well established, the treatment usually requires hot hydrotherapy or castor oil applications followed by thorough connective tissue work (see Figures 103-118).

The purpose is to reduce scar adherence to the chest wall in order to promote better lymph drainage over to the internal mammary nodes (and perhaps to available subclavian node pathways), as well as to enhance the range of motion and therefore the vascular pumping potential of the shoulder joint.

It is also common for women to be encouraged to make a routine of raising their affected side arm over their head (full shoulder abduction) and massaging distal to proximal along the arm to help reduce fluid accumulation. The idea of recommending self massage several times a day to lessen edema build-up is a good one, but anatomically this approach does not entirely make sense. It is more in keeping with flow along the lymph channels to suggest an amendment, namely that she lies supine and holds her arm loosely upwards at a ninety degree angle to the floor (shoulder mid-flexion) and massages distal to proximal in this position. It is also more likely that she will be comfortable with this range of movement earlier than shoulder abduction.

Scar Work

As has already been discussed, breast scars can cause women a number of problems, including pain, reduced range of motion, and obstruction of circulation and drainage. Some scars are also distressing because adhering, pulling, and tension can make them esthetically less pleasing.

Breast scar treatment can offer clients a great deal of improvement, and is very satisfying work for the therapist. The next series of Figures are photographs illustrating scar work.

Figure 100 shows a client with a typical mastectomy scar. In Figures 101 and 102, the therapist is showing adherence of the scar to the chest wall.

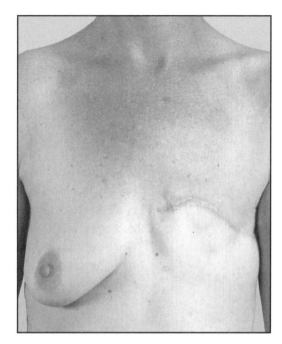

Figure 100

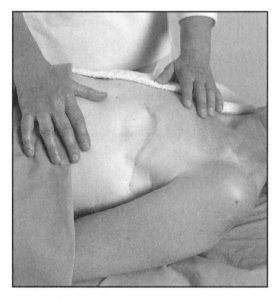

Figure 101

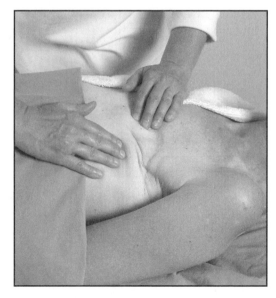

Figure 102

Breast scars are often more adherent or non-compliant with surrounding tissues than might be the norm because of the lack of dissectible surfaces which allow the surgeon to cut and re-arrange tissues along natural lines. As a result there can be a greater tendency for puckering and pulling as the scar dehydrates and 'contracts' within its tissue host. There is also a greater tendency for large planes of adherence to develop.

Since the breast does not have active internal supports like muscles, its fascial membranes take all the stresses of gravity and body activities. When there is an area of tissue scarring or adhering present, these forces can be exerted unevenly. In response to such pressures, breast scars are very susceptible to spreading and bulging, or alternatively, to becoming strongly thickened and reinforced.

Ideally, the massage therapist would like to begin work on optimizing fibre orientation once collagen deposition is well started but the scar has not consolidated (10-14 days). However, in the majority of cases the practitioner is beginning to treat a scar after it has become well established. Because breasts do not have inherent muscles, the exertion of 'good' forces, which ordinarily help a developing scar adjust its collagen fibre direction to the lines of force normal to the body part, does not occur. In fact, bras tend to hold breasts tightly to the chest wall while their scars are forming. Well established scars in the breast often have a non-functional, matted fibre pattern.

In order to promote re-orientation of collagen fibres within a scar, the therapist must first warm and soften the tissue matrix in which the fibres reside. This can be accomplished by the physical forces of manipulation alone, but it is more painful for the client, and since manipulation of breast scarring should be done as much as possible without placing large scale stresses on the supporting fascial membranes, a less aggressive approach is best.

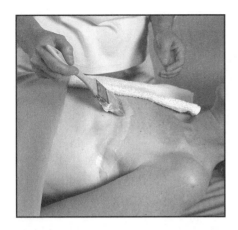

Figure 103

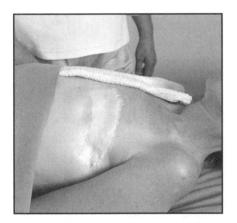

Figure 104

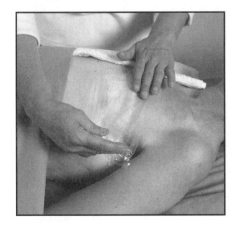

Figure 105

Hydrotherapy is an important tool which can help the tissue reach a more pliable state before manual therapy begins. Figures 103 through 107 demonstrate an approach which can be very effective in getting heat to penetrate into the scar tissue. Using a standard paraffin/mineral oil mix which has been heated to a temperature as hot as maximum skin tolerance, brush several layers directly onto the scar site (Figures 103 and 104). Cover completely with a sheet of plastic (Figures 105 and 106). Next place a hot hydrocollator pack over the treatment area (Figure 107).

The heat penetrates through the wax layer, which acts to both warm up and soften the scar tissue. The plastic prevents easy heat dissipation, causing additional warming and greater penetration of the heat energy into the scar structure. The hot pack should be left on for at least 10 minutes.

There are several other viable approaches which the massage practitioner can utilize. Hot castor oil compresses are excellent for scar work. A cervical hydrocollator pack can be used, with or without wax application, for inframammary scars. The pack is lined up along the bottom edge of both breasts with its curvature placed upward onto the lower aspect of the sternum.

If heat is not appropriate, room temperature castor oil packs can still be quite effective, assuming the client applies them daily at home as well.

Practitioners with advanced training in direct or indirect fascial release techniques will also be able to employ these to great effect, especially if done in conjunction with heat applications.

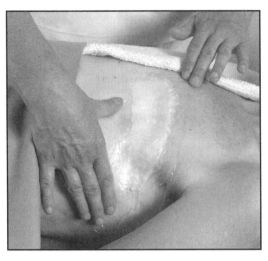

Figure 106

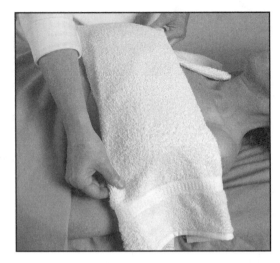

Figure 107

After the pack and paraffin have been removed the skin will feel very soft and there will be hyperemia apparent within the scar. The manual techniques used on-site have no prescribed style or sequence. The goal is to loosen the collagen fibre linkages which have developed within the scar and the adherences between it and its surrounding tissues. The best scar work occurs when the therapist is palpating the matted and 'stuck' elements in the tissues and applying pressures to the specific points and directions of resistance, in other words, concentrating effective force on local areas. Figures 108 through 118 illustrate examples of this type of technique.

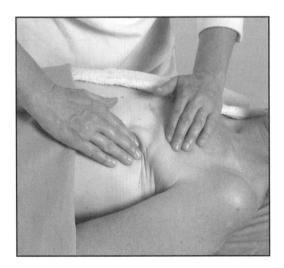

Figure 108

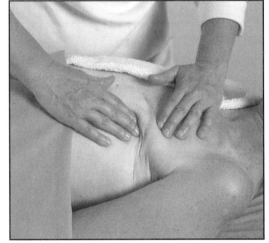

Figure 109

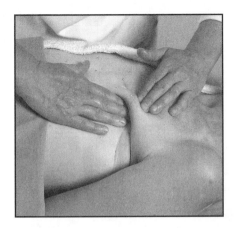

Figure 110

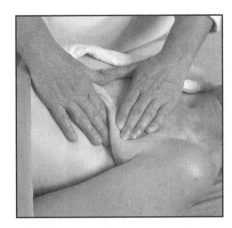

Figure 111

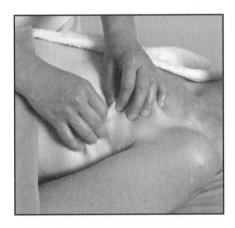

Figure 112

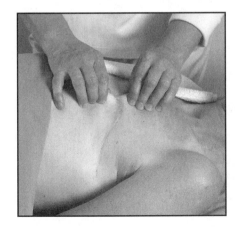

Figure 113

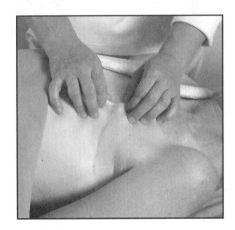

Figure 114

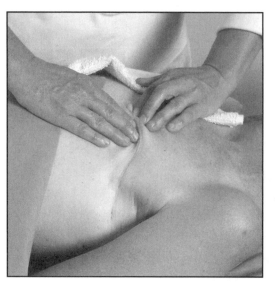

Figure 115

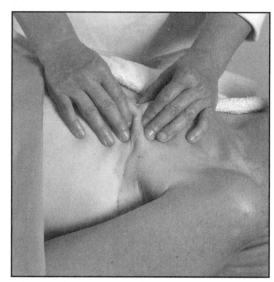

Figure 116

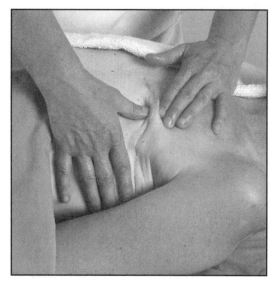

Figure 117

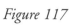

Figure 118

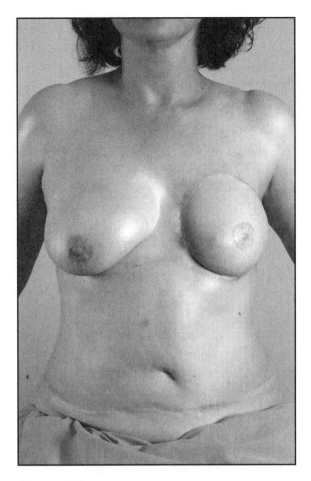

Figure 119

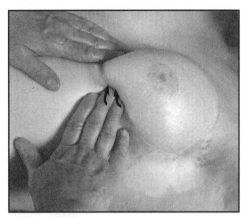

Figure 120

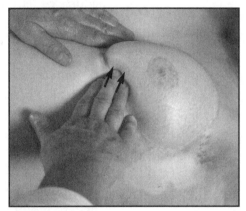

Figure 121

The client in Figures 119-122 has had a rectus abdominis flap (TRAM) operation. Because of radiation damage to her skin, she had the free flap version of the procedure. Bits of this damage can be seen beyond the borders of the grafted skin. Take note of the nicely tattooed nipple.

In Figures 120 through 122, the massage therapist is demonstrating small specific friction techniques on the skin graft scars.

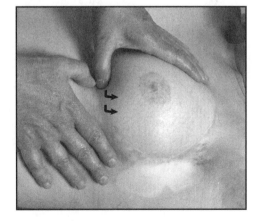

Figure 122

Some Final Notes About Scar Work

1. The massage therapist will often encounter scars that have 'puckers' or areas of tissue which seem to be folded or twisted. Especially common locations in the breast are the 'upturn' sections of inframammary scars in breast reductions, and in mastectomies, a region of tissue just lateral to the sternum. These scar segments are particularly likely to cause pain and to promote collection of pockets of localized swelling. This type of scar formation can be addressed effectively using the modalities already mentioned. Indirect fascial release techniques can be very helpful.

2. Women have a great deal of investment in breast appearance. As a result, breast scars often hold more private emotional significance than scars in other body parts. Breast scarring is also frequently connected to fearful associations with cancer investigation, diagnosis, and treatment. The massage practitioner's approach to breast scar treatment needs to incorporate the added sensitivity and awareness that goes with an understanding of these psychoemotional realm significances. A practitioner who does not feel comfortable working with a client's scars, either technically or emotionally, or does not have sufficient training, should make an appropriate referral to another massage therapist.

3. Like all 'phantom' parts, a breast which has been removed still has a presence for the client, and the sensitivity considerations outlined in this book largely still apply when working with mastectomy scars.

REFERENCES

1. Data in this section condensed from Haagensen, C.D., Chapter 1, "Anatomy of the Mammary Glands", Diseases of the Breast, 3rd edition, W. B. Saunders, 1986

2. Osborne, M.P., "Breast Development and Anatomy", Harris, J.R., Hellman, S., Hendersen, I.C., Kinne, D.W., eds: Breast Diseases, 2nd edition, J.B. Lippincott, 1991, p.4

3. Smallwood, J.A., "The Normal Breast", Smallwood, J.A. and Taylor, I., eds: Benign Breast Disease, Edward Arnold, 1990, p.2

4. The seminal research on this was done by: Turner-Warwick, R.T., "The Lymphatics of the Breast," British Journal of Surgery, 1959, 46:574-582 and replicated by: Hasell, S., Smith, J., Beatlage, C., et al, "Lymphatic Drainage of the Breast by Vital Dye Staining and Radiography", Annals of Surgery, 1965, 162:221-226; reported in Smallwood and Taylor, ibid, p.2

5. Haagensen, C.D., op cit, pp. 27-28. Haagensen is referencing Turner-Warwick as in #4 above.

6. Extensive discussion of this by Haagensen, ibid, pp. 35-39

7. Smallwood, op cit, p.2

8. Haagensen, C.D., op cit, pp. 27-28.

9. Hughes, L.E., Mansel, R.E., Webster, D.J.T., Benign Disorders & Diseases of the Breast, Baillière Tindall, 1989, p. 7

10. ibid, p. 10

11. ibid, p. 12

12. Love, S.M., Gelman, R.S., Silen, W., "Fibrocystic 'Disease' of the Breast. A Non-Disease", New England Journal of Medicine, 1982, 307:1010-1014; referenced in Hughes, Mansel, and Webster, op cit, p. 1

13. ibid, p. 28

14. Ramzy, I., "Pathology of Benign Breast Disease", Mitchell, G.W. Jr., Bassett, L.W., eds: The Female Breast & Its Disorders, Williams & Wilkins, 1990, p. 85

15. Smallwood, op cit, p. 10

16. McCulloch, P. and George, W.D., "Fibroadenosis", Smallwood and Taylor, ibid, p. 59

17. ibid, p. 60

18. World Health Organization, "Histological Typing of Breast Tumours", 2nd edition, 1981, quoted in Hughes, Mansel, and Webster, op cit, p. 59

19. Ramzy, op cit, p. 92

20. ibid

21. ibid, p. 89

22. Hughes, Mansel, and Webster, op cit, p. 95

23. First study: Frantz, V.K., Pickren, J.W., Melcher, G.W., Auchincloss, H., "Incidence of Chronic Cystic Disease in So-Called Normal Breasts", Cancer, 4:762-783, 1951; second study: Foote, F.W., Stewart, F.W., "Comparative Studies of Cancerous Versus Non-Cancerous Breasts," Annals of Surgery, 121:6-53, 1945; both referenced in Hughes, Mansel, and Webster, ibid, p. 94

24. ibid, p. 21

25. Chetty, U., "Nipple Discharge", Smallwood and Taylor, op cit, p. 90

26. Sandison, A.T., "An Autopsy Study of the Adult Human Breast", National Cancer Institute Monograph Number 8, Washington, D.C.: U.S. Department of Health Education Medicine, 1982, pp. 1-45, referenced in Chetty, U., ibid

27. Tedeschi, L.G., Saced, A., Byrne, J.J., "Involutional Mammary Duct Ectasia and Periductal Mastitis", American Journal of Surgery, 106:517-21, 1963; reported in Rogers, K., "Breast Abscesses and Problems with Lactation", Smallwood and Taylor, ibid, p. 100

28. Preece, P.E., "Mastalgia", Smallwood and Taylor, ibid, p. 46

29. Guyer, P.B., "Imaging in Benign Breast Disease", Smallwood and Taylor, ibid, pp. 32-38

30. Rogers, K., "Breast Abscesses and Problems with Lactation", Smallwood and Taylor, ibid, p. 106

31. Newton, E.R., "Lactation and Its Disorders", Mitchell and Bassett, op cit, p. 66

32. ibid, p. 65

33. Gadzhaev, A.C., Legchlo, A.N., "Breast Massage in the Initial Stage of Mastitis is a Cause of Serious Development of the Disease", Klinicheskaia Khirurgiia, Jan/1980, pp. 30-31

34. Ramzy, op cit, p. 83

35. Newton, op cit, p. 66

36. Hughes, Mansel, and Webster, op cit, p. 145

37. Newton, op cit, p. 67

38. Nichols, S., Water, W.E., Wheeler, M.J., "Management of Female Breast Disorders by Southampton General Practitioners", British Journal of Medicine, 281:1450-53, 1980; and Roberts, M.M., Elton, R.A., Robinson, S.E., French, K., "Consultations for Breast Disorders in General Practice and Hospital Referral Patterns," British Journal of Surgery, 74:1020-22, 1987; these sources quoted in: Hughes, Mansel, and Webster, op cit, p. 75

39. Leinster, S.J., Whitehorse, G.H., Walsh, P.V., "Cyclical Mastalgia: Clinical and Mammographic Observations in a Screened Population", British Journal of Surgery, 74: 220-2, 1987; referenced in: Leinster, S.J., "How to Measure Psychological Morbidity in Women with Benign Breast Disease," Mansel, R.E., ed., Recent Developments in the Study of Benign Breast Disease, p. 192, Parthenon, New Jersey, 1992

40. Hughes, Mansel, and Webster, op cit, p. 79

41. ibid, p. 79

42. Terada, S., Tomimatsu, N., Suzuki, N., Kohama, T., Akasofu, K., Nishida, E., "Ultrasonic Changes of Mastopathy Associated with Danazol", Mansel, op cit, p. 32

43. Hughes, Mansel, and Webster, op cit, p. 78

44. ibid, p. 77

45. ibid, p. 78

46. Galea, M.H., Blamey, R.W., "Non-Cyclical Breast Pain: 1-Year Audit of an Improved Classification", Mansel, op cit, p. 79

47. Travell, J.G., & Simons, D.G., "Myofascial Pain & Dysfunction", The Trigger Point Manual, Volume I, The Upper Extremities, pp. 576-597, 344-367, 598-608, and 614-621

48. Smallwood, op cit, p. 9

49. "Benign Breast Disease – An Introduction to the Problem", Smallwood and Taylor, ibid, p. ix 90

50. Chetty, ibid, p. 85

51. Horgan, K., "The Management of Nipple Discharge", Mansel, op cit, pp. 203-204

52. Information derived from Powell, D.E. and Stelling, C.B., The Diagnosis & Detection of Breast Disease, Mosby, St. Louis, 1994, pp. 424-430

53. Brody, G.S., "On the Safety of Breast Implants", Plastic and Reconstructive Surgery, 100(5): 1314-1321, October/97. This incidence estimate is also given in several of the other breast implant sources used.

54. Dumble, L.J., "Dismissing the Evidence: The Medical Response to Women with Silicone Implant-Related Disorders", Health Care for Women International, 17: 515-525, 1996

55. Noone, R.B., "A Review of the Possible Health Implications of Silicone Breast Implants", Cancer, 79(9): 1747-1756, May1/97. Similar estimates are given in several other sources used.

56. McInnis, W.D., "Plastic Surgery of the Breast", Mitchell and Bassett, op cit, p. 196

57. Brody, op cit

58. Gutowski, K.A., Mesna, G.T., Cunningham, B.L., "Saline-Filled Breast Implants: A Plastic Surgery Educational Foundation Multicenter Outcomes Study", Plastic and Reconstructive Surgery, 100(4): 1019-1027, September/97

59. ibid

60. Noone, op cit

61. Brody, op cit

62. Noone, op cit

63. Park, A.J., Black, R.J., Sarhadi, N.S., Chetty, U., Watson, A.C.H., "Silicone Gel-Filled Breast Implants and Connective Tissue Diseases", Plastic and Reconstructive Surgery, 102(2): 261-268, February/98

64. Lewin, S.L., Miller, T.A., "A Review of Epidemiologic Studies Analyzing the Relationship Between Breast Implants and Connective Tissue Diseases," Plastic and Reconstructive Surgery, 100(5): 1309-1313, October/97

65. Giltay, E.J., Bernelot Moens, H.J., Riley, A.H., et al, "Silicone Breast Prostheses and Rheumatic Symptoms: A Retrospective Follow Up Study", Annals of Rheumatic Disease, 53:194, 1994; referenced in Park, et al, op cit

66. McLaughlin, J.K., Fraumeni, J.F. Jr., Olsen, J., Mellemkjaer, L., "Re: Breast Implants, Cancer, and Systemic Sclerosis", Journal of the National Cancer Institute, 86: 1424, 1994, referenced in Lewin and Miller, op cit

67. Hennekens, C.H., Lee, I.-M., Cook, N.R., et al, "Self-Reported Breast Implants and Connective Tissue Diseases in Female Health Professionals: A Retrospective Cohort Study", Journal of the American Medical Association, 275: 616, 1996; referenced in Park et al, op cit

68. Hodgkinson, D.J., Letters Section, Medical Journal of Australia, 166(2): 615-616, June 2/97

69. Dumble, op cit

70. Young, V.L., Riolo Nemecek J., Schwartz, B.D., Phelan, D.L., Watson Schorr, M., "HLA Typing in Women with Breast Implants", Plastic and Reconstructive Surgery, 96(7): 1497-1519, December/95

71. Teuber, S.S., Rowley, M.J., Yoshida, S.H., Anasri, A.A., Gershwin, M.E., "Anticollagen Antibodies are Found in Women with Breast Implants," Journal of Autoimmunity, 6: 367, 1993; referenced in Young et al, op cit

72. Wall, W., Martin, L., Frittzler, M.J., Edworthy, S., "Non-Fasting Chylomicroanaemia in Breast Implant Recipients", The Lancet, Letters to the Editor section, 345: 1380; referenced in Dumble, op cit

73. Ellis, T.M., Hardt, N.S., Campbell, L., Piacentini, D.A., Atkinson, M.A., "Cellular Immune Reactivities in Women with Silicone Breast Implants: A Preliminary Investigation", Annals of Allergy, Asthma, and Immunology, 79: 151-154, August/97

74. Noone, op cit

75. Brody, op cit

76. Noone, op cit

77. Brinton, L.A., Malone, K.E., Coates, R.J., Schoenberg, J.B., Swanson, C.A., Daling, J.R., Stanford, J.L., "Breast Enlargement and Reduction: Results From a Breast Cancer Case-Control Study", Plastic and Reconstructive Surgery, 97(2): 269-275, February/96

78. Kern, K.A., Flannery, J.T., Kreehn, P.G., "Carcinogenic Potential of Silicone Breast Implants: A Connecticut Statewide Study", Plastic and Reconstructive Surgery, 100(3): 737-747, September/97

79. Brody, op cit

80. Levine, J.J., Ilowite, N.T., Pettei, M.J., Trachtman, H., "Increased Urinary NO3- + NO2- and Neopterin Excretion In Children Breast Fed by Mothers with Silicone Breast Implants: Evidence for Macrophage Activation", Journal of Rheumatology, 23(6): 1083-1087, 1996

81. Mathes, S.J., "Editorial: Breast Implantation – The Quest for Safety and Quality", New England Journal of Medicine, 336(10): 718-719, March 6/97

82. Huang, T.T., "Breast and Subscapular Pain Following Submuscular Placement of Breast Prostheses", Plastic and Reconstructive Surgery, 86(2): 275-280, August/90

83. Vinnik, C.A., "Spherical Contracture of Fibrous Capsules Around Breast Implants: Prevention and Treatment", Plastic and Reconstructive Surgery, 58: 555, 1976; referenced in Melmed, E. P., "Treatment of Breast Contractures with Open Capsulotomy and Replacement of Gel Prostheses with Polyurethane-Covered Implants", Plastic and Reconstructive Surgery, 86(2): 270-274, August/90

84. Melmed, ibid

85. McInnis, op cit, p. 200

86. Gabriel, S.E., Woods, J.E., O'Fallon, W. M., Beard, C.M., Kurland, L.T., Melton, L.J., "Complications Leading to Surgery after Breast Implantation", New England Journal of Medicine, 336(10): 677-682, March 6/97

87. Adams, J.P. Jr., Robinson, J.B. Jr., Rohrich, R.J., "Lipid Infiltration as a Possible Biologic Cause of Silicone Breast Implant Aging", Plastic and Reconstructive Surgery, 101(1): 64-71, January/98

88. Beckman, W.H., Feitz, R., Hage, J.J., Mulder, J.W., "Lifespan of Silicone Gel-Filled Mammary Prostheses", Plastic and Reconstructive Surgery, 100(7): 1723-1726, December/97

89. Noone, op cit

90. Brody, op cit

91. Noone, op cit

92. Peters, W., Smith, D., "Calcification of Breast Implant Capsules: Incidence, Diagnosis, and Contributing Factors", Annals of Plastic Surgery, 34(1): 8-11, January/95

93. Wallace, M.S., Wallace, A.M., Lee J., Dobke, M.K., "Pain After Breast Surgery: A Survey of 282 Women", Pain, 66: 195-205, 1996

94. ibid

95. Huang, op cit

96. Roberts, C., Wells, K., Daniels, S., "Outcome Study of the Psychological Changes after Silicone Breast Implant Removal", Plastic & Reconstructive Surgery, 100(3): 595-599, September/97

97. Godfrey, P.M., Godfrey, N.V., "Response of Locoregional and Systemic Symptoms to Breast Implant Replacement with Autologous Tissues: Experience in 37 Consecutive Patients", Plastic & Reconstructive Surgery, 97(1): 110-116, January/96

98. ibid

99. Polseno Crawford, D., "Why Don't We do Breast Massage?", Massage Therapy Journal, 36(4): 94-106, Winter, 1998

100. Curties, D., "Breast Massage: Discussion Paper and Suggested Guidelines", Journal of Soft Tissue Manipulation, 1(1): 4-6, June/July, 1993

101. Fitch, P., "The Case for Breast Massage", Massage Therapy Journal, 36(4): 64-78, Winter, 1998

102. Polseno Crawford, D., op cit

103. ibid

104. Small, E., "Psychology and Psychopathology in Breast Disorders", Mitchell and Bassett, op cit, p. 75

105. Extensive coverage in: Harris, D.R., "Healing of the Surgical Wound", Parts I & II, Journal of the American Academy of Dermatology, 1 (3): 197-215, September/79

106. Allen, M., Oberle, K., "Augmentation Mammoplasty: A Complex Choice", Health Care for Women International, 17: 81-90, 1996

107. Yamamoto, Y., Nohira, K., Sugihara, T., Shintomi, Y., Ohura, T., "Superiority of the Microvascularly Augmented Flap: Analysis of 50 Transverse Rectus Abdominis Myocutaneous Flaps for Breast Reconstruction", Plastic & Reconstructive Surgery, 97 (1): 79-83, January/96

108. Schnur, P.L., Schnur, D.P., Petty, P. M., Hanson, T.J., Weaver, A.L., "Reduction Mammoplasty: An Outcome Study", Plastic & Reconstructive Surgery, 100 (4): 875-883, September/97

BIBLIOGRAPHY

Annals of Allergy, Asthma, and Immunology

- Ellis, T.M., Hardt, N.S., Campbell, L., Piacentini, D.A., Atkinson, M.A., "Cellular Immune Reactivities in Women with Silicone Breast Implants: A Preliminary Investigation", 79: 151-154, August/97

Annals of Plastic Surgery

- Dowden, R.V., "Achieving a Natural Inframammary Fold and Ptotic Effect in The Reconstructed Breast", 19(6):524-9, 1987

- Peters, W., Smith, D., "Calcification of Breast Implant Capsules: Incidence, Diagnosis, and Contributing Factors", 34(1): 8-11, January/95

Barth, V. & Prechtel, K., **Atlas of Breast Disease**, B.C. Decker Inc., 1991

Cancer

- Noone, R.B., "A Review of the Possible Health Implications of Silicone Breast Implants", 79(9): 1747-1756, May 1/97

Cawson, R.A., McCracken, A.W., Marcus, P.B., Zaatori, G.S., **Pathology: The Mechanisms of Disease**, 2nd ed., C.V. Mosby, Co., 1989

Drever, J.M., "Natural Breast Tissue Reconstruction and Augmentation", Patient Hand-Out Information

Haagensen, C.D., **Diseases of the Breast**, 3rd ed., W.B. Saunders, 1986

Handchirurgie, Mikrochirurgie, Plastische Chirurgie

- Volvmallinck, H.E., "Long Term Results Following Breast Augmentation" (trans.), 16(2): 118-121, June/84

Harris, J.R., Hellman, S., Henderson, I.C., Kinne, D.W., **Breast Diseases**, 2nd ed., J.B. Lippincott, 1991

- Osborne, M.P., "Breast Development and Anatomy"

Health Care for Women International

- Allen, M. & Oberle, K., "Augmentation Mammoplasty: A Complex Choice", 17: 81-90, 1996

- Dumble, L.J., "Dismissing the Evidence: The Medical Response to Women with Silicone Implant-Related Disorders", 17: 515-525, 1996

Hughes, L.E., Mansel, R.E., Webster, D.J.T., **Benign Disorders and Diseases of the Breast**, Baillière Tindall, 1989

Journal of the American Academy of Dermatology

- Harris, D.R., "Healing of the Surgical Wound", Parts I & II, 1(3): 197-215, September/79

Journal of Rheumatology

- Levine, J.J., Ilowite, N.T., Pettei, M.J., Trachtman, H., "Increased Urinary NO3-+NO2- and Neopterin Excretion In Children Breast Fed by Mothers with Silicone Breast Implants: Evidence for Macrophage Activation", 23(6): 1083-1087, 1996

Journal of Soft Tissue Manipulation

· Curties, D., "Breast Massage: Discussion Paper and Suggested Guidelines", 1(1): 4-6, June/July, 1993

Journal of Surgical Oncology

· Zanolla, R., Monzeglio, C., Balzarini, A., & Martino, G., "Evaluation of the Results of Three Different Methods of Postmastectomy Lymphedema Treatment", 26(3):210-3, 1984

Klinicheskaia Khirurgiia

· Gadzhaev, A.C., Legchlo, A.N., "Breast Massage in the Initial Stage of Mastitis is a Cause of Serious Development of the Disease" (trans.), pp.30-31, January/1980

Kumar, V., Cotran, R.S., Robbins, S.L., **Basic Pathology**, 6th ed., W.B. Saunders, 1997

Love, S.M., **Dr. Susan Love's Breast Book**, 2nd ed., Addison-Wesley, 1995

Mansel, R.E., **Recent Developments in the Study of Benign Breast Disease**, Parthenon Publishing Group, 1992

· Galea, M.H. & Blamey, R.W., "Non-Cyclical Breast Pain: A 1-Year Audit of an Improved Classification"

· Gately, C.A., Miers, M., Skona, J.F., Mansel, R.E., "The Cardiff Mastalgia Clinic Experience of the Natural History of Mastalgia"

· Horgan, K., "The Management of Nipple Discharge"

· Leinster, S. J., "How to Measure Psychological Morbidity in Women with Benign Breast Disease"

· Terada, S., Tomimatsu, N., Suzuki, N., Kohama, T., Akasofu, K., Nishida, E., "Ultrasonic Changes of Mastopathy Associated with Danazol"

Massage Therapy Journal

· Fitch, P., "The Case for Breast Massage", 36(4): Winter, 1998

· Polseno Crawford, D., "Why Don't We Do Breast Massage?", 36(4): Winter, 1998

Medical Journal of Australia

· Hodgkinson, D.J., Letters Section, 166(2): 615-616, June 2/97

Mitchell, G.W. Jr., & Bassett, L.W., **The Female Breast and Its Disorders**, Williams & Wilkins, 1990

· Beller, F., "Development and Anatomy of the Breast"

· Farber, M., Chhibber, G., Hewlett, G., "Medical Management of Benign Breast Disease"

· McInnis, W.D., "Plastic Surgery of the Breast"

· Mitchell, G.W. Jr., "Ambulatory Surgery for Diagnosis and Treatment"

· Newton, E.R., "Lactation and Its Disorders"

· Ramzy, I., "Pathology of Benign Breast Disease"

· Small, E., "Psychology and Psychopathology in Breast Disorders"

Netter, F.H., **Atlas of Human Anatomy**, Novartis, 1989

New England Journal of Medicine

· Gabriel, S.E., Woods, J.E., O'Fallon, W.M., Beard, C.M., Kurland, L.T., Melton, L.J., "Complications Leading to Surgery after Breast Implantation", 336(10): 677-682, March 6/97

· Mathes, S.J., "Editorial: Breast Implantation - The Quest for Safety and Quality", 336(10): 718-719, March 6/97

Pain

- Wallace, M.S., Wallace, A.M., Lee, J., Dobke, M.K., "Pain After Breast Surgery: A Survey of 282 Women", 66: 195-205, 1996

Pelton, R., Clarke Pelton, T., Vint, V.C., **How to Prevent Breast Cancer**, Simon & Schuster, 1995

Plastic and Reconstructive Surgery

- Adams, J.P. Jr., Robinson, J.B.Jr., Rohrich, R.J., "Lipid Infiltration as a Possible Biologic Cause of Silicone Breast Implant Aging", 101(1): 64-71, January/98
- Barnett, G.R., Carlisle, I.R., Gianoutsos, M.P., "The Cephalic Vein: An Aid in Free TRAM Flap Breast Reconstruction: Report of 12 Cases", 97(1): 71-78, January/96
- Barnett, G.R., Gianoutsos, M.P., "The Latissimus Dorsi Added Flap for Natural Tissue Breast Reconstruction: Report of 15 Cases", 97(1): 63-70, January/96
- Becker, H. & Prysi, M.F., "Quantitative Assessment of Postoperative Breast Massage", 86(2):355-6, August/90
- Beckman, W.H., Feitz, R., Hage, J.J., Mulder, J.W., "Lifespan of Silicone Gel-Filled Mammary Prostheses", 100(7): 1723-1726, December/97
- Brinton, L.A., Malone, K.E., Coates, R.J., Schoenberg, J.B., Swanson, C.A., Daling, J.R., Stanford, J.L., "Breast Enlargement and Reduction: Results From a Breast Cancer Case-Control Study", 97(2): 269-275, February/96
- Brody, G.S., "On the Safety of Breast Implants", 100(5): 1314-1321, October/97
- Godfrey, P.M., Godfrey, N.V., "Response of Locoregional and Systemic Symptoms to Breast Implant Replacement with Autologous Tissues: Experience in 37 Consecutive Patients", 97(1): 110-116, January/96
- Gutowski, K.A., Mesna, G.T., Cunningham B.L., "Saline-Filled Breast Implants: A Plastic Surgery Educational Foundation Multicenter Outcomes Study", 100(4): 1019-1027, September/97
- Huang, T.T., "Breast and Subscapular Pain Following Submuscular Placement of Breast Prostheses", 86(2): 275-280, August/90
- Kern, K.A., Flannery, J.T., Kreehn, P.G., "Carcinogenic Potential of Silicone Breast Implants: A Connecticut Statewide Study", 100(3): 737-747 September/97
- Lewin, S.L., Miller, T.A., "A Review of Epidemiologic Studies Analyzing the Relationship Between Breast Implants and Connective Tissue Diseases", 100(5): 1309-1313, October/97
- Melmed, E.P., "A Review of Explantation in 240 Symptomatic Women: A Description of Explantation and Capsulectomy with Reconstruction Using a Periareolar Technique", 101(5): 1364-1371, 1998
- Melmed, E.P., "Treatment of Breast Contractures with Open Capsulotomy and Replacement of Gel Prostheses with Polyurethane-Covered Implants", 86(2): 270-274, August/90
- Park, A.J., Black, R.J., Sarhadi, N.S., Chetty, U., Watson, A.C.H., "Silicone Gel-Filled Breast Implants and Connective Tissue Diseases", 102(2): 261-268, February/98
- Roberts, C., Wells, K., Daniels, S., "Outcome Study of the Psychological Changes after Silicone Breast Implant Removal", 100(3): 595-599, September/97
- Schnur, P.L., Schnur, D.P., Petty, P.M., Hanson, T.J., Weaver, A.L., "Reduction Mammoplasty: An Outcome Study", 100(4): 875-883, September/97

- Yamamoto, Y., Nohira, K., Sugihara, T., Shintomi, Y., Ohura, T., "Superiority of the Microvascularly Augmented Flap: Analysis of 50 Transverse Rectus Abdominis Myocutaneous Flaps for Breast Reconstruction", 97(1): 79-83, January/96

- Young, V.L., Riolo Nemecek, J., Schwartz, B.D., Phelan, D.L., Watson Schorr M., "HLA Typing in Women with Breast Implants", 96(7): 1497-1519, December/95

Powell, D.E. & Stelling, C.B., **The Diagnosis and Detection of Breast Disease**, C.V. Mosby Co., 1994

Smallwood, J.A., & Taylor, I., **Benign Breast Disease**, Edward Arnold, 1990

- Chetty, U., "Nipple Discharge"

- Dixon, J.M., "Cystic Disease of the Breast"

- Guyer, P.B., "Imaging in Benign Breast Disease"

- Hobby, J.A.E., "Plastic Surgery Techniques for Non-Malignant Breast Disease"

- McCulloch, P. and George, W. D., "Fibroadenosis"

- Preece, P.E., "Mastalgia"

- Rogers, K., "Breast Abscesses and Problems with Lactation"

- Smallwood, J.A. & Taylor, I., "Benign Breast Disease - An Introduction to the Problem"

- Smallwood, J.A., "The Normal Breast"

Travell, J.G. & Simons, D.G., **Myofascial Pain and Dysfunction, The Trigger Point Manual, Volume I, The Upper Extremities**, Williams & Wilkins, 1983

INDEX

boundaries, 120; psychoemotional reactions, 116, 122–23, 133, 147, 167, 194

client-therapist relationship. *See* therapeutic relationship

closed capsulotomy, 86–87

collagen, 36

collagen capsule, 84

collagen deposition, 47, 184

collagen membrane capsule, 24

collecting duct, 18*f*

colostrum, 34, 35

communication, client-therapist, 124–26, 127–31, 140–41; guidelines, 146–47; non-verbal, 127–29; pre-consent, 133; role-play scenarios, 141; training, 139, 140–41

connective tissue (CT) disease, 75–80

consent, informed, 123, 132–34, 142; guidelines, 146–47; renewal, 133, 147

contraindications for treatment, 105

Cooper's ligaments, 18*f*, 106

costochondritis, 62

cyclical mastalgia, 60

cysts, 17, 36, 47–50*f*, 64, 65*f*, 171*f*; lipid, 53; micro-, 36, 47

diabetes, 53, 56, 66, 68, 179

dopamine antagonist drugs, 64

drainage tubes, 173*f*, 181

draping, 142–46*f*, 148, 158; full undraping, 142; massage through sheet or clothing, 144*f*; regulations concerning, 143

Dressed to Kill (Singer and Grismaijer), 32

duct, 18*f*, 25*f*

duct channels, 26

duct ectasia, 50–52*f*, 53, 56, 61, 64, 107

duct inflammation, 50

ductules, 25*f*, 26

dysesthesia, 92, 107, 183

dysplasia, 63

edema, 181, 185–86

effleurage techniques, 156–58*f*, 163, 185

epithelial hyperplasia, 42

epitheliarization, 180

esophageal lesions, 62

estrogen, 41, 44–45, 60

external mammary nodes, 30*f*, 31

fascial membranes, 106

fascial release techniques, 187–94

fibroadenoma, 43–45*f*, 65*f*

fibroadenosis, 42–43*f*, 60

fibrocystic breast disease, 40, 41

fibrosis, involutional, 64

figure-8 wrap, 169

foreign body mastitis, 56

gall stones, 62

gel bleed, 70

general treatment protocols, 123

glandular epithelial cells, 24, 26

glandular epithelium, 25*f*

glandular function, 33

glandular system, 24–25

guidelines, 110, 135, 146–50, 179–86

gynecomastia, 68

heart attack, 62

heart infections, 62

heat applications, 189–90

hematoma, 53, 181, 185

hiatus hernia, 62

hormonal functions, 26, 33

hormonal imbalance, 41, 43, 64, 68

hormone replacement therapy, 49, 60

human adjuvant disease, 75

human leukocyte antigens (HLAs), 78

hydrotherapy, 55, 58, 185, 189–90*f*

hygiene concerns, 169, 180, 181

immune system, 30; autoimmune diseases, 56, 75, 78; reaction to silicone, 73–75

implants, 16, 69–93; anticollagen antibodies, 79; for breast augmentation, 90, 174; calcification, 88, 89; capsule contracture, 84–87, 89, 90, 93; cause of abscess, 53; cause of mastitis, 56; clinical problems, 83–93; closed capsulotomy, 86–87; connective tissue (CT) disease, 75–80; contraindications for massage, 105; extrusion, 93; fibrous capsules, 86; fill seepage, 70–71, 88;

gel bleed, 71; guidelines, 149; historical background, 70–73; immunological reaction, 73–75; incisions for, 172*f*; link with cancer, 81; lipid abnormalities, 79; migration, 91; obsolescence, 107, 149; pain, 61, 84, 88, 89–92; paraffin injection, 89; placement, 85*f*, 86, 90, 91–92, 173*f*; post-surgical issues, 83–84, 89–92; removal, 92–93; rupture, 86, 87–88; saline, 72–73, 89; sensory abnormalities, 92; shell, 70; silicone, 70–72*f*, 73–80; silicone injection, 53, 70, 89

incisions, 171*f*, 172*f*, 173*f*, 178*f*, 184–85

indications for breast massage, 104

infection, 56, 105, 185

inflammatory autoimmune conditions, 56

inflammatory diseases, 53, 56

informational resources, 131, 146

inframammary incision, 172*f*, 173*f*

inframammary scars, 189, 193

intercostal arteries, 26

intercostal muscles, 155*f*

intercostal nerves, 33

intercostobrachial nerve, 33

internal mammary artery, 26

internal mammary nodes, 30*f*, 185–86

internal mammary vein, 27*f*

internal thoracic blood vessels, 31

internal thoracic nodes, 31

interpectoral nodes, 30*f*, 31

intramammary lymph node, 53

involution, 17, 36–37

involutional fibrosis, 64

ischemia, 106, 181, 185

ischemic pain, 91

lactation, 17, 35–36, 61, 107, 170; after breast reduction surgery, 178; breast changes during, 35–36*f*; hygiene concerns, 169; lactational mastitis, 54–56, 169; massage during, 167–70; nipple damage, 54; problems with breast implants, 82

lactiferous sinus, 18*f*, 25*f*

laser endoscopy, 85

latissimus dorsi, 22

latissimus dorsi flap, 176–77*f*

legislation and regulation, 110, 143

ligaments of Cooper, 18*f*, 106

lipid cyst, 53

lipoma (in males), 68

lobe, 24, 25*f*

lobular involution, 47

lobules, 18*f*, 24

lumen obstruction, 47

lump, 16; description, 135; discovery of, 39, 95, 134–36; mobility, 64–65*f*; ominous characteristics, 64–65; undiagnosed, 105, 134–36

luteal phase, 60

lymphatic drainage, 28–31*f*, 32, 148, 151, 162; for breast abcess, 58; for lactational mastitis, 55; for post-mastectomy edema, 186; stimulation of channels, 152*f*

macrocysts, 36, 47–50*f*

macrophages, 73–74

male breast conditions, 68, 106

male therapists, 95, 117–18, 146

mammary, 16

mammary dysplasia, 41

mammogram, 45*f*, 48*f*

massage therapists: attitudes to breast massage, 39, 95–96, 99–100, 103; avoidance of area surrounding breast, 103; choice to avoid breast massage, 98–99, 108, 115, 125, 139, 147; choice to avoid scar work, 194; consultation with physicians, 179–80; discovery of abnormalities, 39, 63, 134–36; guidelines for, 147–48; male, 95, 117–18, 146; power differential, 111; self-awareness, 111–16; sexual misconduct, 97, 99, 109, 117–18, 119

mast-, 16

mastalgia, 16, 59–62

mastectomy, 16, 172–74; breast reconstruction, 85, 90, 173*f*, 174; cancer recurrence, 81; chronic pain, 90; hydrotherapy for scar, 185, 189–90*f*; phantom limb phenomena, 107, 149, 194; post-surgical edema, 185–86; scar adherence, 186, 187*f*; skin puckering, 194; standard procedure, 173*f*

mastitis, 16, 53, 54–59; bacterial, 35, 57; foreign

body, 56; lactational, 54–56, 59, 105, 169; non-lactational, 56–57; viral, 56
menopause, 36, 49, 60
menstrual cycle, 36, 40–41, 42, 45, 59–60
microcysts, 36, 47
milk, 24, 35, 107, 170
milk sinus, 25
mobilization: of breast tissue, 159–64*f*; of shoulder, 164
Montgomery's glands, 20
myocutaneous flaps, 92–93, 175–77
myoepithelium, 26, 34
myofascial trigger points, 62

needle aspiration of macrocyst, 50*f*
nerve(s), 33; damage, 182; nerve-related pain, 90, 91, 182; nerve root compression, 33
nipple, 18*f*, 20*f*; accessory, 22; avoidance of, 144, 151, 162*f*; damage during lactation, 54; discharge from, 17, 46, 50, 51, 63–64; lymph drainage, 28; macrocysts behind, 49–50; nerve supply, 33; pigmentation, 34; retraction, 51, 64, 107; sexual response, 20, 33; tattooed (after reconstruction), 173, 177, 193*f*; tenderness and pain, 35, 52, 54, 91
non-cyclical mastalgia, 61–62

ominous signs, 17

pain: in arm, 91, 183; from duct ectasia, 52; from implants, 61, 84, 88, 89–92; ischemic, 91; from macrocysts, 49–50; mastalgia, 16, 59–62; musculoskeletal origins, 33, 106; nerve-related, 90, 91, 182; post-surgical, 89–92, 182–83; psychosomatic, 62; from sclerosing adenosis, 46
painful nodularity, 42
pain referral, 106
palpation of lumps: fibroadenoma, 43; fibroadenosis, 42; macrocysts, 48–49; ominous lump, 64–65; sclerosing adenosis, 45–46
paraffin injection, 89
paraffin treatment, 189
paraesthesia, 107, 183
parenchyma, 24–26, 25*f*, 28, 35
peau d'orange, 66*f*

pectoral (anterior axillary) nodes, 30*f*
pectoral fascia, 18*f*, 29*f*
pectoralis major, 18*f*, 19, 22, 29*f*, 31, 62, 86, 170; removal with mastectomy, 172; treatment and relaxation, 148, 151, 153–54*f*
pectoralis minor, 31, 62, 170
peer supervision groups, 114
periareolar incision (for implant), 172*f*
perimenopause, 36
petrissage techniques, 159–64*f*, 185
pleurisy, 62
post-surgery, 83–84, 179–86; edema, 181, 185–86; fatigue, 183; guidelines, 107, 149, 179–86; hygiene concerns, 180; observation of site, 182; pain, 89–92, 182–83; sensory abnormalities, 182, 183–84. *See also* scars and scar tissue; surgery
pregnancy: breast changes during, 34–35; breast massage during, 167–70; fibroadenoma enlargement, 45; position adaptations, 168*f*; problems with breast implants, 82
professional issues, 108; association with sex trade, 95, 98; role of breast massage, 98–99; supervision relationships, 114
progesterone, 41
psychotherapy, 114, 119, 137

quadrant system of landmarking, 23*f*

rectus abdominis, 22; lymphatics, 30*f*, 31; TRAM procedure, 175–76*f*, 193*f*
referrals, 108, 118, 136–37; to physicians, 134, 137, 182, 183
regulations, 110, 143
retromammary space, 18*f*, 19, 29*f*
rib, prominent, 53
ribcage asymmetry, 53
Rotter's nodes, 30*f*, 31

scalenes, 62, 170
scapular nodes, 30*f*
scars and scar tissue, 61, 171–78*f*, 185. *See also* post-surgery; surgery
scar work, 169, 187–94*f*
sclerosing adenosis, 45–46, 60